Stories From The Field

A History of Wilderness Therapy

Will White

Stories From The Field:

A History of Wilderness Therapy

Will White

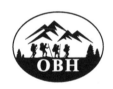

Wilderness Publishers
Jackson, New Hampshire

wildernesspublishers.com

Copyright

Stories From The Field: A History of Wilderness Therapy

First paperback edition published in the United States of America, October, 2015

ISBN-10: 0-692-51243-8   ISBN-13: 978-0-692-51243-2

10   9   8   7   6   5   4   3   2   1

For permission requests to reproduce selections from this book, write to the publisher, subject line: Attention: Permissions Coordinator:
wild@wildernesspublishers.com

Colophon: This book is set in Garamond, Garamond Bold, Garamond Italic, Garamond Bold Italic. The text is set, 12/14.4 x 28.

All profits from this book go to research.

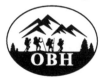

Wilderness Publishers
PO Box 155
Jackson, NH 03846

wildernesspublishers.com

for
Adam Tsapis

Table of Contents

Acknowledgments

This book is dedicated to Adam Tsapis. I am grateful to have had Adam as a friend and business partner at Summit Achievement for almost twenty years. Adam passed away on February 16, 2015 in a kite skiing accident before the completion of the book. He had read several chapters and encouraged me to continue writing this book when I just wanted to walk away. He was a good man, a good father, a good friend. I miss you Adam and this book is for you. Hope you like it.

I am grateful to my wife Lisa White, and our two sons Caleb and Micah, who have been a great support during the years I worked on this book. They encouraged me while keeping it into perspective.

I am grateful to Patrick Logan (Launch IT) with his amazing powers to correct grammatical errors and question different paths in the first half of the book. Many a time I turned around and went another direction after talking with Patrick.

I am grateful to Bonnie Richardson, Nichol Ernst, Jake Weld, Carl Lovejoy, Thom Pollard, Heilan Yvette Grimes, Gil Hallows, Dr. Lee Gillis, Dr. Keith Russell, Dr. Anita Tucker, and Dr. Joanna Bettman Schaefer for reading and reviewing and giving feedback on the book before publication.

I am grateful to Gary Ferguson for all he has done to share the story of the field and for writing the foreword of this book.

If it was not for all of the following contributing writers and their programs, the second half of this could not have come into being. I am grateful to all of the following people and their programs who contributed in putting the second half of this book together. They are truly the storytellers of the histories of their programs. Contributors to this collection are Steve Glass (Project D.A.R.E. – Wendigo Lake), Bev Oldham (Enviros), Matt Claybaugh (Marimed), Ezekiel Sanchez (Anasazi), Sean Hoyer and John Conway (Omni Youth Services – Journey), Kumen Jones (RedCliff Ascent), Gil Hallows (Outdoor Behavioral Healthcare Council, Legacy Outdoor Adventures), Lorri Hanna and Doug Sabo (Soltreks), Devan Glissmeyer and Cheryl Kehl (Second Nature), Mike Gass, Anita Tucker and Maggie Karoff (Outdoor Behavioral Healthcare Research Cooperative), Rebecca Vines (SUWS of the Carolinas), Rick Meeves (Outback Therapeutic Expeditions), Rob Meltzer (Wilderness Therapy Symposium), Suzanne McKinney (Pacific Quest), Mod Barefoot (True North Wilderness Program), Aaron Fernandes (Open Sky Wilderness Therapy), John Karren and Andrew Powell (Elements), Jess Shade (Aspiro Adventures), Drew Hornbeck and Steve Sawyer (New Visions), Shayne Gallagher (Wingate), Brian Johnson (Trails Carolina), Beth Fogel (Expedition Therapy), Lynnette Spencer (Adventure Works), Madolyn Liebing (The Journey and The Achievement Foundation) and Rick Heizer (Evoke Therapy Programs).

I am grateful for the support from all of the people involved with Summit Achievement over the years and especially the spring and summer of 2015. I am grateful to the other co-founders of Summit Achievement, Chris Mays, Candide Kane, Andy Richardson, thank you for inviting me on this journey.

To Tobie Feigenbaum, Eben Tsapis, Ezra Tsapis and Noa Tsapis, Kyra Gould and the rest of the Tsapis family – thank you for sharing Adam with me.

To my parents, Joan and Marcus White, thank you for encouraging me to go to summer camp and being in Boy Scouts (even though I did not always appreciate it). Your love of wild places helped guide me to this field.

I am grateful to the all the families who trust this field with their children. Thank you.

Foreword

It's hard to imagine a more reliable set of clues to the essence of human spirit, than to consider that which has long been shimmering though our relationships with the natural world. Time and again we've learned, forgotten, and then learned all over again how nature can be a prompt for learning to live well in the world – urging us not to escape life, but to more fully embrace it. And over the past many decades, no group has done more to help us not just consider such truths, but actually live them, than the practitioners of wilderness therapy.

In the spring of 1998 I had the great good fortune of experiencing wilderness therapy first hand, spending four months at a program in southern Utah's canyon country for a book I was writing called *Shouting at the Sky*. By then I was already familiar with the idea of nature as healer. But living day to day in that astonishing place, amidst what were incredibly creative people, I began to see that the success of wilderness therapy was derived less from "treating" individuals per se, than from employing nature as a means of releasing both innate talents, as well as the capacity for self authority. Perhaps more notable still, once such growth ignited, it tended to be quickly followed by an eager desire to serve the community.

I came to believe that this urge to be generative, to establish what amounts to a healthy, beneficent personal ecology, happened as fast as it did because of the wild setting where we resided. Perhaps it was simply that nature offers the two essential prompts that have long been considered essential for human transformation journeys – one being sacred time, and the other, sacred space. But whatever the reason, it was the wilderness part of wilderness therapy that seemed to really anchor conscious growth – offering students and staff alike a daily nourishment of presence and gratitude and humility.

Seven years after that experience, in 2005, it was me who was broken, struggling in the wake of having lost my wife and wilderness companion of twenty-five years, Jane, in a canoeing tragedy in northern Ontario. Overwhelmed by sadness, one day I decided to get in touch with some of the students I'd come to know at that program in southern Utah. One was working as an accountant, another a history professor. There were two nurses, a chef. Also an oil rig foreman, an advertising executive, a furniture builder, a financial planner. We talked about how nature had been so good at bringing us back to the present moment, even at those times when we were trying our best to run away. We talked about the cycle of losing and finding, of things ending and then beginning again. We recalled how great it felt to need each other.

In this wonderful chronicle of wilderness therapy, Will White offers a thoughtful, much-needed touchstone to the evolution of what is arguably one of the most extraordinarily effective mental health efforts in modern history. As you'll see in these pages, over time such programs have become stronger, safer, and more effective – refinements that in recent years especially have been guided by a tremendous commitment to quantitative research.

Yet for all that, there seems much about this healing model that remains beyond strict analysis. One of the reasons wilderness therapy has succeeded so well is because those involved have been willing at various turns to be as original, unruly, and creatively audacious as nature itself. Those who serve the practice best are those who continue to insist that room be made for the ineffable flow of mystery, for that dazzling alchemy that can happen when we bring a sense of beauty to the honoring of each other's pain. If practitioners can remain humble in the face of their considerable success, willing to not just to seek answers but to practice living with questions – and further, if they can continue to insist that wild nature be the ground that gives life and nourishment to their efforts – then wilderness therapy will likely continue for many years to be a precious wellspring of strength and healing.

The history recounted in these pages is part and parcel of America's long, passionate love affair with nature. A relationship that has informed to an incredible degree our sense of who we are; and at the same time, a canvas onto which we easily imagine that which we might yet be. Thanks to *Stories From The Field,* wilderness therapy can now begin to take its place in this compelling national story – encouraging us toward some greater personal authenticity, toward the realization of a stronger, more heartfelt unity between us and this exquisite world in which we live.

Gary Ferguson
Red Lodge, Montana

Preface

This book is a story of stories. It is a story of experiences about people, places, and things, many of which are interconnected and have shaped the evolution of wilderness therapy. This story begins with a story of how I came to weave this book together. I could say it was my childhood being sent to wilderness therapy programs every summer (it was summer camp but it was therapeutic for me) and being forced by my parents into a paramilitary training organization to teach me self discipline and outdoor survival (it was Boy Scouts and it did teach me self discipline), but those stories would make this preface too long.

So I will start this story by saying that it was a fortuitous combination of a manuscript review followed by a mid-life crisis. In 2007, I was asked by an editor and some authors to look over a book manuscript about the field of wilderness therapy, as I had been in the field for over twenty years, had co-founded a wilderness therapy program (Summit Achievement), and held different leadership positions in professional organizations related to the field. The majority of the book was quite useful but the chapter about the history of wilderness therapy was lacking in depth and breadth and so I encouraged the editor and authors to develop the genealogy of wilderness therapy.

The history chapter was not expanded and it bothered me as there is so much to this field. Although my ego was bruised, I quickly moved on as I was too busy acting out the aforementioned mid life crisis.

My mid-life crisis, at least that is what my wife and friends called it, was enrolling in a doctoral degree program at the spry age of 47. At different times during the graduate degree process, each of us thought it would have been easier on us all if I had just bought a sports car or began doing triathlons.

While pursuing my doctorate, I found myself focusing my class projects on the history of the wilderness therapy field. In a research class I interviewed leading practitioners and academicians from the field of wilderness therapy about the origins of the field and found that there were widely differing views as to the early influences. I discovered that all the documented histories of the field were very limited in breadth, exclusive to a short span, a few programs or restricted to a particular model or philosophy. But as an active participant in the field, I have heard the web of oral histories recounted at conferences and workshops, tales of the various social and political inflections, the pioneers and personalities, and the proud and turbulent evolution of wilderness therapy. It seemed a shame, and an error, that no one had provided a comprehensive history of the field. I decided to take on the task of writing a history of the field for my dissertation. My dissertation was titled "Stories from the Elders: Chronicles and Narratives from the Early Years of Wilderness Therapy," (available at http://gradworks.umi.com/35/05/3505069.html).

My second round of writing about the history of the field came when I was invited by leading researchers in the field, Drs. Mike Gass, Lee Gillis, and Keith Russell, to contribute a history chapter for their book, *Adventure Therapy: Theory, Research, and Practice.* With that, I compressed much of my doctoral research into a summation of the evolution of the field. After the book was published and dissertation completed, I presented my research at numerous conferences. During those presentations, I received feedback from attendees about what I missed or misrepresented.

And alongside the history, I was encouraged to include modern day programs. I was interested in updating my research but was concerned, as many modern-day wilderness therapy programs were founded by contemporaries, friends, and/or competitors. Another challenge was the only histories available were marketing websites and those were generally limited in their scope. This lack of objective content tempered my enthusiasm.

One weekend I was camping with my family and my epiphany came when we were all sitting around a campfire at the end of the day and my children were telling stories. The stories they were telling were stories from their summer adventures. My children's stories are theirs and not mine. It was during that campfire story telling session that I decided to ask founders or current leaders in wilderness programs to write their stories about their program's founding and evolution – from their viewpoint. To help inspire people to tell their stories, I asked them to write and donate their stories for the good of the field and without the expectation of any financial remuneration. I received 26 chapters; stories from the different people weaved into a history of wilderness therapy for the good of the field with all profits going to research. I am grateful to all of the contributors (see Acknowledgments section)

The book is a comprehensive chronicle of the history of the wilderness therapy field and narratives from present day wilderness therapy organizations. The book is formatted in two sections: Part I is titled "A Chronicle of the Evolution of Wilderness Therapy," and includes a literature review that identifies organizations and influences that emerged from 1860-1960, and a literature review that identifies organizations and influences that emerged from 1961 to the present. Part II is titled "Narratives from Present Day Programs." This section includes the 26 present-day narratives.

How to Read this Book

I encourage you to take your time with this book. First spend time reading and, perhaps, rereading the chronicle section and letting the foundation sink in. There is a great deal of information in this document. The chronicle section reviews some of the controversies in the field. Much of what has happened, like any history, is not pretty. History is not clean or simple. Some of you will read the chronicle section and think I reviewed too many of the controversies. Others will think that I did not review enough. Some may think I missed some pieces and others may say I was too inclusive. I agree with all of you. Each of us interprets history through our own biases and, although I worked on keeping an eye on my biases, I know it was not perfect. Nothing is. This is "a" history, not the complete history of wilderness therapy. That would take volumes and while writing those books, more volumes would emerge, as history is always moving. My hope is that it is enough of the history so that others will be inspired to add to it whether it is good, bad, or ugly.

When reading the narrative section I encourage you to either literally, or figuratively, place yourself under the stars, around a campfire and surround yourself with the stories of how this fascinating, profound and varied treatment philosophy developed.

Part I

A Chronicle of the Evolution of Wilderness Therapy

"If you don't know history, it's as if you were born yesterday"

– Howard Zinn

It could be said that wilderness therapy is first documented in Biblical writings in the Book of Genesis with Ishmael and Hagar being banished to the wilderness. Others may argue that it could be traced to indigenous tribes in a ceremony in which young people were sent out into the wilderness to fend for themselves in order to formalize the transition from adolescence to adulthood. However, it is not the intent of this book to identify the actual genesis of wilderness therapy, but to chronicle and illuminate the numerous influences that have helped shape this evolving behavioral healthcare field. At its core, the history of wilderness therapy is about organizations and leaders who have operated outside of the mainstream of behavioral healthcare and/or education – the visionaries whose wild and unconventional ideas proved indispensable to the success of students, families and programs today. This first section provides a chronological presentation of early organizations, leaders, and events that influenced the evolution of the field.

And from whence did wilderness therapy spring? What were the impetus and needs that spawned the early programs to reimagine the field, to cleave away from traditional treatments and set out on what seemed so radical a course at the time? This evaluation will begin by identifying the organizations and leaders that first integrated the use of the outdoors for character development or as a rehabilitative and recuperative tool for young people in order to explore the many influences that have helped shape, inform, and define wilderness therapy as it is seen today. These organizations and leaders are cited in articles, books, on-line documents and, in some instances, personal communication, in order to fill in missing pieces. This Historical Perspective section will: a) reveal the extensive history of the use of the out-of-doors for character development and treatment of young people in the United States; b) reveal the history of controversies related to outdoor programs for youth; and c) cite connections between organizations. Identified throughout are critical books, articles, and peripheral professional organizations related to the field.

To provide a chronological organization, each program will be identified by start date, leaders and their background influences, as well as ideas and practices. There are a few facts to be mindful of when reading this section. It should be noted that each organization listed influenced the field in significant ways (though not always for the better). It is also important to note that this historical review is focused on wilderness therapy for youth; although it does include some organizations which serve young adults, it should not be seen as encompassing all wilderness treatment organizations for adults, which has its own unique story.

This historical perspective of wilderness therapy is divided into Chapter 1 and Chapter 2. Chapter 1 is titled "Foundation: The Camping Movement" as it chronicles the first organizations, primarily camps, that have incorporated outdoor experiences to impact youth, character and behavior, from 1861 to 1962. Chapter 2 is titled "Transformation: From Wilderness Survival to Wilderness Therapy to Outdoor Behavioral Healthcare." As the title suggests, it chronicles organizations that initially called themselves wilderness survival programs, then wilderness therapy programs, and have more recently, specifically from 1962 – 2012, developed an accreditation and structure as outdoor behavioral healthcare organizations.

Chapter 1

The First Hundred Years
1860-1962: Foundation
The Camping Movement

T HE ORIGINS OF WILDERNESS THERAPY CAN BE traced back to the 1800s when organized camping for youth emerged in the United States. Organized summer camps were first developed by educators from Northeast boarding schools and universities in order to address the unstructured summer months of wealthy American youth. These educators were seen as "radical" by other educators during their time, as they were interested in influencing youths' behavior through outdoor living experiences (Eells, 1986). These educators were not focused on academics but the broader skills of adulthood and character development, especially the dignity, and value, of work.

Psychiatrist Elton McNeil (1957), in his article "The Background of Therapeutic Camping," explained that camping was always about therapy for young people. McNeil attributed the development of the first summer camps to the idea that "deeply rooted in our cultural conception of mental hygiene (health) for the developing child has always been the view that 'idleness' or 'undirected activity' is destructive to 'character'" and so declared that "an orderly program of 'character building' activities, under the supervision of model adults, was the essential pattern of camping in its early days" (p. 3). McNeil stated that organized camping evolved as an antidote to the physical and moral decline of youth due to the changing industrial society and its movement towards mechanization and urban living. With impressive prescience, McNeil (1957) predicted that more therapeutic camp programs would emerge and that mental health "trained professionals" would become more involved (p. 11). He felt that more research would be needed to evaluate the "effectiveness of therapeutic efforts" in wilderness settings (p. 10).

McNeil's reflections on the early influences of therapeutic camping are affirmed by the first organized summer camps. The first organized summer camps originated in New England, the first at The Gunnery, while the second organized summer camp, Camp Chocorua, marks the beginning of practices that would shape future thinking in the field of organized camping and, eventually, wilderness therapy.

1861: The Gunnery

Fredrick William Gunn founded The Gunnery in Washington, Connecticut in 1850, enrolling girls, international students and students of color. Gunnery Camp, the first summer camp for youth was organized in 1861, according to Eleanor Eells (1986), camp director, college professor and historian, in her book, *History of Organized Camping: The First 100 Years.* Gunn, an educator, prominent abolitionist, and outdoorsman, "believed that vigorous hiking and year-round sports strengthened not merely muscle, nerve, and self-discipline, but developed a masculine character" (p. 5). The students at The Gunnery were eager to live their romanticized view of a soldier's life, which included camping under the stars (this was during the Civil War). Gunn also saw value in a summer school term in the outdoors so, in August of 1861, he and his wife took the entire school on a two-week hiking and camping trip (p. 5). Gunn continued the summer camp until 1879. It should be noted that Gunn also had a pragmatic objective for his summer school session. This objective is one of sustainability and consistency and included continued collection of tuition payments from parents and the ability to keep working with students during the summer months. (The Gunnery no longer runs a therapeutic/character development summer camp but still operates a boarding school and summer sports at its original location.)

The second organized summer camp did not start as an adjunct to a boarding school but started with the intention of changing the behavior of wealthy American boys. The name of the organization was Camp

Chocorua and its founder proposed using outdoor experiences to change adolescent behaviors.

1881: Camp Chocorua

Camp Chocorua opened in 1881 on Burnt Island on Squam Lake in New Hampshire. According to Eells (1986), Camp Chocorua was founded by Ernest Balch, a deeply religious man and Dartmouth College student, who developed strong opinions on the perils of wealthy American youth. Balch was one of eight children who grew up on a New Hampshire farm and actively participated in the daily job of putting food on the table. Balch also knew a great deal about living in the woods. Upon entering Dartmouth College, he encountered wealthy young men who had not developed the same work-related value system, nor did they have any knowledge of the outdoors. Balch developed the camp in order to combat "the miserable existence of wealthy adolescent boys in the summer when they must accompany their parents to fashionable resorts and fall prey to the evils of life in high society" (p. 7). Balch wanted campers to become "responsible, independent, and resourceful" and so there "would be no servants, no class distinctions, and no snobbery" at this small camp (p. 7). The camp did not have a mess hall or cooks, and all meals were cooked by campers over an open fire. Every camper had to learn how to swim, sail, and paddle a canoe in any type of weather. Not only were outdoor skills essential but Balch believed that each boy should learn the value of money in a capitalist society. Therefore each boy had a twenty-five cents per week allowance that they earned by doing chores. The camp ran like a small community with a church, bank, court system and camp newspaper. Not only did the camp have an intricate system in place to develop responsibility in campers, it also established written objectives referred to as the Camp Chocorua Principles.

The Camp Chocorua Principles focused on "1) the development of a sense of responsibility in the boy, both for himself and others, and 2) appreciation of the worthiness of work" (Eells, 1986, p. 8). These principles, and Camp Chocorua's lack of affiliation with any school, led to Ernest Balch's reputation as the "father of the organized camping movement" (Eells, 1986). Ideas of addressing the overindulgence of youth with time in the out-of-doors and increasing self-responsibility for young people via time in the wilderness are ideas that originated at

Camp Chocorua with Ernest Balch. Camp Chocorua closed after eight years. Balch was no longer interested in his camp once he had proven the value of the camp experience to other educators. Ernest Balch would be contacted throughout his life by other educators, camp founders, and directors as to his theories and experiences in running Camp Chocorua.

A majority of the early summer camps used the Camp Chocorua principles as an outline for their organizations. This includes the first summer camp for girls only, Camp Arey, which was located in Arey, New York. It is worthy to note that, in 1915, Balch did continue his work with camps, developing, in association with the Cloyne School, the first winter camp program occurring during Cloyne's winter breaks.

The Camp Chocorua organization and its leader, Ernest Balch, were critical in the evolution of wilderness therapy. It was the beginnings of the organized summer camp movement which would eventually include campers with psychological issues. Chocorua was also the first organization that intentionally utilized outdoor living with the express intention that adolescent participants would become "responsible, independent, and resourceful" young adults. Balch's ancestors still spend summers on Squam Lake and his great grandnephew, Will Twombly, would follow his ancestor's work in the field as a clinician in several different wilderness therapy programs, including Catherine Freer Wilderness Therapy, Pacific Quest, and True North Wilderness Program. It was from these utilitarian beginnings of the organized summer camp movement that programs would eventually include and even specialize in campers addressing their psychological issues in the wilderness milieu.

During the late 1800s and 1900s, organized summer camps flourished in the United States and around the world. It was in 1901 that the first use of the outdoors to treat mental illness would occur, but purely by accident.

1901: Manhattan State Hospital

Psychologist Ruth Caplan (1974), in the book *Camping Therapy*, revealed that during the summer of 1901 amidst a tuberculosis outbreak, Dr. A. E. Macdonald, superintendent of the Manhattan State Hospital (an "insane asylum"), placed forty psychiatric patients, with tuberculosis, in tents on the facility grounds in order to separate them from non-tubercular patients. Caplan described the hospital staff being so impressed with the psychological and physical improvement of the tent patients that twenty non-tubercular psychiatric patients were also placed in tents on the grounds. A majority of those patients improved, some to the point of being discharged. She adds that, by the end of the summer, most of the remaining patients were placed back into the building whereby they showed marked regression, while a small group of seriously ill tubercular patients, who were placed in a winterized tent, continued to show improvement (p. 9). She describes that the "tent treatment" occurred again at the hospital the following spring and summer and patient improvement continued. What started as a way to address the tuberculosis outbreak unintentionally resulted in fewer psychological and physical symptoms in diverse patients, where the only variable was time in the outdoors.

According to Caplan (1974), "Tent Treatment" became a minor fad in institutions during the early 1900s, and its course may best be traced to Manhattan State Hospital's "half-yearly summaries of hospital events in the *American Journal of Insanity*" (p. 10). She adds that "tent treatment" did not retain its standing for long. Its real value, the small group, was eliminated for the purpose of increasing patient census and the original tents were replaced with rustic frame structures (p. 10). Her concluding paragraph states that, by the early 1920s, journal articles about camp treatment came to a halt and the use of camping for treatment "slipped out of sight until it was rediscovered in the late 1950s and early 1960s" (p.12). Her concluding paragraph is accurate in the case of adults with mental illness, but inaccurate in relation to adolescents (information that may be easier to discover because of current research technology). Numerous articles and documents, related to adolescent therapeutic camps, were published in the 1920s, '30s, and '40s, some of which will be reviewed later in this section.

The rich compilation of articles in *Camping Therapy* (1974), edited by psychologist Thomas Lowry, focuses primarily on adult mental health institutions in the 1960s, and the integration of camping and its inherent wilderness living skills into the adult treatment milieu. Before revealing these first organized camps specifically for psychologically challenged youth, it is important to review The Boy Scouts of America, an organization that has placed more youth in the wilderness than any other, and has influenced the structures, models and many founders of today's wilderness therapy programs.

1907: The Boy Scouts

The Boy Scouts was founded in 1907 in England by Lieutenant-General Robert Baden-Powell, a war hero and author, according to retired psychiatrist and Scout leader Edward Rowan (2005) in his book *To Do My Best: James E. West and the History of the Boy Scouts of America.* Baden-Powell, an advisor to the British Empire, recognized that young men from urban British neighborhoods did poorly in the military as they had no outdoor skills and little respect for authority. Baden-Powell wanted to "do something to improve the character of boys" so he developed a "comprehensive scheme for boy training" (Rowan, 2005, p. 24). In August of 1907, he brought an economically diverse group of twenty-two boys for a two-week camping experience on Brownsea Island, in the Southern tip of England. The purpose of this experience was to teach them outdoor skills, character education, and military training. The experience was then written up and published in 1908 as a book titled *Scouting for Boys,* which became quite popular in England. In 1910, Baden-Powell retired from the military to work full time promoting scouting in Britain and abroad. After numerous requests from girls seeking programs, Baden-Powell started Girl Guides, later known as Girl Scouts in the United States, with organizational support from his sister Agnes Baden-Powell in 1910.

1910: Boy Scouts of America

Boy Scouting was brought to the United States in 1910 by William D. Boyce, a wealthy American publisher and world traveler. Boyce had a chance encounter in London in 1909 with an unknown Boy Scout who offered to help him cross a busy street (Rowan, 2005). So impressed by the boy's refusal of a tip, Boyce learned all he could about Scouting and brought the organization to the United States. Boyce incorporated the Boy Scouts of America in 1910 but he did not have the time or platform to make the organization grow. Shortly thereafter, Boyce had a meeting with Edgar M. Robinson, the Secretary for the International Department of the Young Men's Christian Association (YMCA), to discuss ways to expand Scouting in the United States. "Robinson was always looking for ways to get boys into his (YMCA's) buildings, in order to get their attention and mold their character. For Robinson and YMCA leaders throughout the world, the Boy Scouts' scheme was an ideal way to do that" (Rowan, 2005, p. 29). Robinson approached Boyce suggesting that the YMCA would be a good organization to help promote the Boy Scouts movement in America. Boyce turned the organization over to Robinson who opened the first Boy Scouts of America (BSA) office in June of 1910 at a YMCA in New York City. With the financial support of Boyce, the Boy Scouts was delivered through YMCA affiliates rapidly spreading across the United States (Rowan, 2005).

Two other men, Ernest Seton and Daniel Beard, were also critical to the evolution of Boy Scouting. Seton, an author and naturalist, developed the Woodcraft League for Boys in 1902 after his house in Connecticut was vandalized by local boys (Rowan, 2005). The Woodcraft League was an outdoor program that consisted of "tribes" of boys who practiced Native American primitive outdoor skills learned from Seton's book, *The Birchbark Roll* (Rowan, 2005). Seton met Baden-Powell in 1906 and gave him a copy of *The Birchbark Roll*. As the author of the first *Boy Scouts Handbook* and the first BSA Chief Scout, Seton was influential in the adoption of Native American primitive skills by the BSA (Rowan, 2005). In 1905, Beard, a naturalist, artist, and devout Christian, founded the Sons of Daniel Boone to expose boys to nature and to "instill the spirit of the pioneers" (Rowan, 2005, p. 26). Beard folded the Sons of Daniel Boone into the BSA, founded the first Scout Troop (Troop 1), and was a National Scout Commissioner for thirty years (Rowan, 2005). All the men involved in the early days of the Boy Scouts in America and Britain had "a common goal – to develop character in boys" (Rowan, 2005, p. 30).

Boy Scouts of America (BSA) was one of the earliest and largest organizations to utilize the out-of-doors to help develop character of adolescents. Scouting, with its origination from Baden-Powell, a military man, is a hierarchal program with badges in which scouts can earn ranks (Tenderfoot to Eagle). To move up through the rankings, a scout must master skills in order to obtain merit badges, each rank progressing in woodcraft and hard skills and leadership ability to the highest level, Eagle Scout. According to the BSA website, "The BSA provides a program for young people that builds character, trains them in the responsibilities of participating citizenship, and develops personal fitness" (Boy Scouts of America, 2011). According to the facts published by the BSA, 56% of United States astronauts were involved in Scouting, and 35% of West Point cadets were involved with Scouting. In addition, 15% of West Point cadets were Eagle Scouts (the highest rank achieved by less than 5% of Boy Scout participants). Obviously, Scouting is an incredibly popular, successful, and impactful program, but the BSA has had its share of controversies.

One of the controversies in Boy Scouting has been the incidents of sexual abuse by volunteers, which was initially concealed by the National Scout Organization. Patrick Boyle (1994), in his book, *Scouts Honor: Sexual Abuse in America's Most Trusted Institution,* posits "scouting has always been a magnet for men who are sexually attracted to boys" (p. 20). In the early years (i.e. 1911), the BSA developed a "Red Flag list" to address this; the list was comprised of names of ineligible volunteers due to allegations of sexual abuse to Scouts. Unfortunately the BSA did not share this information with authorities until the 1980s, which allowed perpetrators to continue this behavior outside of Scouting, or change their names and join a different troop to find additional victims. This tactic, of not involving authorities when a child is being sexually abused by an adult, is similar to the sexual abuse scandals and cover-ups by the Catholic Church in America. In the 1980s, the BSA attempted to address this issue by developing a "Youth Protection Guidelines" video and requiring all leaders and volunteers to watch it (Boyle, 1994). The video reviewed rules for Scout leaders, including rules that mandated one should never let a Scout be alone with an adult and required leaders to report suspicion of abuse. The Youth Protection Guidelines obligated that abuse be reported not only to Scout leaders, but to local authorities. After the development of the Youth Protection Guidelines video and pamphlets, there was a drop in reported sexual abuse. Currently all volunteers and staff involved in Scouting must go through a criminal background check and trainings. This is similar to the majority of modern wilderness therapy programs.

Another controversy that continues to challenge the BSA is its refusal to allow gay men to participate. In a sign of potential political/ethical shifting at the very top of the organization, the Boys Scouts of America released a statement in May, 2013 that announced "today, following this review, the most comprehensive listening exercise in Scouting's history, the approximate 1,400 voting members of the Boy Scouts of America's National Council approved a resolution to remove the restriction denying membership to youth on the basis of sexual orientation alone" (Boy Scouts of America website). However, BSA continues to prohibit adult leaders who are gay, lesbian, or transgender, as well as forbidding volunteers who are atheists. In June of 2000, the United States Supreme Court upheld a ban on gays and atheists as Scout volunteers. According to Chief Justice William H. Rehnquist, the First Amendment's protection for freedom of association meant that the state could not compel the 6.2-million Boy Scouts of America "to accept members where such acceptance would derogate from the organization's expressive message" (Greenhouse, 2000, p. A1). The prohibition of homosexuals and atheists by BSA, and the history of sexual abuse incidents by volunteers, are two of the most prominent controversies associated with the BSA. (Note that as this book was heading to print, the BSA was reconsidering the stance.)

While acknowledging these schisms, it is important to state that the BSA is the largest and most successful volunteer organization focused on character development for adolescents in the United States. The BSA helps to get more young people into the outdoors than any other single organization in the United States (Eells, 1986). The year 2010 was the 100th anniversary of Boy Scouting in the United States.

Chuck Sudetic a journalist with *Rolling Stone Magazine*, reported in 2000 that the Church of Jesus Christ of Latter Day Saints (LDS), informally known as Mormons, is the largest sponsor of Boy Scout troops in the United States and that a large percentage of LDS youth and parents are involved in the organization. As will be revealed in this section, many individuals who influenced wilderness therapy are also members of the LDS church. Many of those individuals involved with wilderness therapy were also associated with Scouting as youth (in the case of full disclosure, this writer achieved the Eagle Scout rank in 1977, but is not a member of the LDS Church).

One of the ways Scouting has influenced the field can be seen in the level system used by many wilderness therapy programs by which participants must master certain skills in order to move up to the next level. This is similar to the rank system of the BSA. One example of this was evidenced at Aspen Achievement Academy (AAA), which was located in Utah. AAA was the oldest wilderness therapy programs in Utah before its closure in 2011 (see next chapter). The highest level a student in AAA could attain was Eagle, a striking similarity with Boy Scouting. In order to make the Eagle level at Aspen Achievement Academy, a student had to not only show individual leadership, academic initiative and therapeutic compliance, but also master many primitive outdoor skills such as long hikes, night travel, self-reliance regarding campcraft, and the consistent ability to make fire with a bow drill. The use of iconic Native American skills and rituals, first implemented by the Boy Scouts of America, continues to be used in many wilderness therapy programs today.

Boy Scouts of America's influence on Wilderness Therapy

Scouting's influence on wilderness therapy seems quite clear. Scouting was the first organization for adolescents to use a level or ranking system to mark the progress of their participants. BSA was the first to integrate primitive survival skills into its curriculum, later adopted by many wilderness therapy programs. BSA opened its first summer camp in 1912 which, second to Camp Chocorua, was one of the earliest to focus on character development. These contributions of the Boy Scouts can also be traced directly to influencing two other major organizations in wilderness therapy's history: Outward Bound USA and Brigham Young University's 480 Class: "Youth Rehabilitation through Outdoor Survival Class." (Both of these organizations will be investigated later in this section.)

1921: Camp Ahmek

One of the most cited books about "therapeutic camping" (Davis-Berman & Berman 1994, 2008; Lowry, 1974) is *Camping and Character* by Hedley Dimock and Charles Hendry (1929). Dimock and Hendry (1929), two social scientists, tell of Camp Ahmek as the first camp that documented and structured the program with the mission of promoting character education for campers. They elaborated that Camp Ahmek was established in 1921 with two primary goals: 1) a recreational function to improve the physical health of campers and; 2) a social function in order to improve the interpersonal skills of campers. They described the Camp as being focused on participants building healthy relationships with other campers in a group setting where camp counselors provided consistent role modeling. *Camping and Character* (Dimock & Hendry, 1929) is an important book to the field of wilderness therapy as it elaborates on the philosophical outlines of therapeutic work with campers. Yet *Camping and Character* (1929) is an in-depth account of therapeutic work with "normal campers" and so its original ideas can be traced back to Ernest Balch and the Camp Chocorua Principles or to Boy Scouting. Similar to Camp Chocorua, Camp Ahmek is, and always has been, focused on "normal" campers and not those with psychological issues. Camp Ahmek is still in existence today and is located in Algonquin Park, Canada.

Indeed Camp Ahmek was considered by some to be a critical organization in the evolution of wilderness therapy. However, it is now clear that Camp Chocorua, the first camp with character development as a goal, was the source of the ideas and the philosophy behind organized summer camps for emotional growth, therapeutic or not. Camp Ahmek carries significance because it is the subject of *Camping and Character* (Dimock & Hendry, 1929), and this book has been useful to both organized camping and therapeutic camps.

Before exploring other organizations, it is pertinent to identify the emergence of therapy as a goal in camps that started in the 1920's and specifically enrolled emotionally challenged young people. Several of the following camps, some of which are still in existence, have not been identified in previous histories of the wilderness therapy field.

1922: Camp Ramapo

The first summer camp developed specifically for emotionally challenged young people was founded in 1922. Joseph Galkin (1937), a psychiatric social worker, observed that Camp Ramapo opened in upstate New York with the specific purpose of working with "delinquent and problem children" (p. 474). The camp was "sponsored by an independent committee of interested and influential men" and was affiliated with the Jewish Board of Guardians, an agency concerned with the treatment of behavior and personality problems of children and adults (p. 474). Camp Ramapo had accommodations for 120 boys who were all in active treatment with the Jewish Board of Guardians. Camp Ramapo's staff, at that time, included psychiatric social workers and counselors. Camp Ramapo still operates today in Rhinebeck, NY, but is now referred to as Ramapo for Children. The organization provides services to male and female "children ages 6 to 16 who are affected by social, emotional, or learning challenges, including children affected by autism spectrum disorders" (Ramapo for Children Website, 2014). Ramapo for Children is the longest running therapeutic camp in the United States.

1935: Camp Wediko

In a 1939 article, titled "An Evaluation of a Psychiatric Camp for Children," Eleanor Cockerill and Helen Witmer, two social workers from Smith College, reviewed the history of the Psychiatric Clinic of the Massachusetts General Hospital Camp. This camp was founded by Dr. Robert Young in 1935. An increase in the budget of the Camp, in 1936, made it possible to rent a completely equipped camp located in the foothills of the White Mountains in Maine. The staff included two psychotherapists, a psychiatrist, who also served as the camp physician, and a psychologist, who served as the camp director. All were staff at the Psychiatric Clinic of the Massachusetts General Hospital and had previously treated children who would become campers. The Camp also had ten counselors who helped run the general camp. The Camp ran for two sessions: one for boys during the month of July and the other for girls during the month of August. According to a doctoral dissertation by Jill Galbraith (1963), the Camp closed during World War II but reopened as the Province Lake Camp in 1948, again under the continued guidance of Dr. Young. Province Lake Camp was later renamed Camp Wediko when it moved to a 450-acre site in Windsor, New Hampshire. Camp Wediko, now referred to as Wediko Children's Services, currently provides services year-round, including a therapeutic school, support services in school settings, and home-based services. Wediko Children's Services continues to operate its summer camp for behaviorally challenged youth and is the second longest running therapeutic camp for adolescents in the United States.

1944: University of Michigan Fresh Air Camps

Dr. William Morse (1947), a psychology professor, wrote extensively about the University of Michigan's Fresh Air camps. These camps initially started in 1921 as summer camps for boys with "inadequate backgrounds" and then transitioned to being a camp specifically focused on working with "maladjusted children" in 1944. In an article titled "From the University of Michigan Fresh Air Camp: some problems with therapeutic camping," Morse (1947) argued that therapeutic camps are more effective for "maladjusted youth" than residential institutions. He offered three reasons: 1) wilderness camp environment provides structure that is not as controlling or artificial as an institution; 2) the camp environment is relaxed without punitive discipline; and 3) the environment allows the therapist to observe the child in an actual relationship with peers, adults, and nature. He also reviewed that the outdoor activities allow for a reduction of tension, permit creative learning without the classroom, and give campers the opportunity to have significant adventures without reverting to antisocial activities. Morse (1957) followed up, ten years later, on the changes in the University of Michigan Fresh Air Camp in an article entitled "An interdisciplinary therapeutic camp." He observed that the Camp moved away from volunteers and had "a staff of counselors composed of about fifty university students who are registered for academic credit in a highly specialized training program" (p. 15). He reviewed that the program evolved to have a professional therapeutic team of a psychologist, sociologist, social worker, pediatrician, and a consulting psychiatrist who helped to oversee the running of the camp and supervise staff and campers. This program appears to be the most clinically sophisticated therapeutic camp of its day and was ahead of its time with the inclusion of a multidisciplinary treatment team. The camp closed in the 1970's because of declining enrollment.

1946: Dallas Salesmanship Club Camp

Camp Woodland Springs, later renamed the Dallas Salesmanship Club Camp, was founded in 1946 with the explicit goal of treating boys with emotional problems. The Dallas Salesmanship Club Camp was directed by Campbell Loughmiller, who earned a B.A. in philosophy, a certificate in social work, and a Master's in Education. Loughmiller, like Ernest Balch, grew up on a family farm with a strong work ethic and commitment to his church. He wrote two books about his experiences at the Dallas Salesmanship Club Camp, one titled *Wilderness Road* (1965) and the other titled *Kids in Trouble* (1979), that are now widely regarded as classics in the field.

From the outset, the Dallas Salesmanship Club Camp had a strong group focus in which the camper was responsible for his own well-being as well as his group's well-being. In *Wilderness Road* (1965), Loughmiller noted that the Dallas Salesmanship Club (not the camp) was founded in 1921 by a group of influential and wealthy men who were active in business and civic life in the Dallas Area. The Dallas Salesmanship Club founders were devoted to the operations of the Camp and all its activities.

Loughmiller described some of the elements of the Dallas Salesmanship Club Camp as follows: "we find the camp environment good because it accords more fully the child's nature and provides ample opportunity to satisfy the desire most boys have for adventure and exploration in the out-of-doors. The small group living in this environment encourages original experimentation and provides the widest possible variety of direct experience with the natural surroundings" (p. 1). Loughmiller did not specifically define therapeutic camping, yet states "therapy is where you find it: and as we see here at camp, it accrues from the many specific procedures as well as from the milieu itself" (p. 123). Although the campers resided in the campgrounds for the majority of the time, on occasion, they would go on three to six week canoe or raft expeditions with their counselors. It was on one of these multi-day raft trip expeditions that two boys from the Camp drowned when their raft capsized. These river expeditions were some of the earliest documented multi-day wilderness trips, outside of a camp setting, with psychologically challenged young people, and sadly, the accidental deaths of participants on these expeditions are some of the earliest documented deaths in therapeutic outdoor programs.

In *Kids in Trouble* (1979), Loughmiller reviewed the type of camper enrolled at the Dallas Salesmanship Club Camp: "All kinds of boys come – aggressive, delinquent, neurotic, schizophrenic; with brain damage, asthma, epilepsy, dyslexia and so on: but as we see it, they are not sick and we are not *therapists*" (p. 22). He also reviews the staff structure at the Camp: "We have no specialists: no psychologists, no psychiatrist, no water-front man, no special teachers. Our services are channeled as fully as possible through the two counselors in charge of each group. This requires that we provide continuous on-the-job training of counselors, because three separate disciplines have their confluence in the daily life of the group: social work, education, and camping" (p. 25). Loughmiller elaborated that the setting of the Camp was far enough away from civilization that there were few distractions. The facilities at the Camp were minimal, only a kitchen and dining hall, bathhouse, warehouse, and office. Each group of boys and their leaders (called "Chiefs") built their own shelters, latrines, and fire pits for cooking. About a third of the meals were cooked at the shelter-site with the rest provided at the dining hall.

Significantly, the Camp also had a strong family focus with regular sessions that parents of campers would have to attend. "The full involvement of parents throughout a boy's stay is the best insurance we have found against post-camp regression" (p. 33). Bolstered by a study done by the University of Texas, Loughmiller summarized the effectiveness of the Camp, stating that, "eighty-five percent of the boys who leave the camp are able to lead responsible and successful lives" (p. 33).

The Dallas Salesmanship Club Camp is a significant organization, for it was the first camp that worked year-round with psychologically challenged young people who would spend a year or more at the camp. Loughmiller (1979) was one of the first to identify the power of the relationship between camper, counselor, and group and recognize that "we are not therapists treating boys with an illness; we are friends helping boys with problems – problems that manifest themselves in ways that are obvious to everyone in the group" (p. 25). Loughmiller and the Dallas Salesmanship Club Camp have been cited as the foundation of many of the wilderness therapy programs in existence today (Davis-Berman & Berman, 2008). Later in life, Loughmiller became focused on photographing the wildflowers of Texas and was the past president of the Texas Chapter of the Nature Conservancy. Loughmiller and his wife, Lynn, coauthored several books, including *Texas Wildflowers: A Field Guide* (2006), *Big Thicket Legacy* (2002), and a book that reveals their devotion to Christianity, *Let's go Camping: Camping and Christian Growth* (1959). Loughmiller died in 1993 and The Dallas Salesmanship Club Camp was closed in 2004, because of budget difficulties, after almost sixty years of helping young people.

The Dallas Salesmanship Club Camp modeled resourcefulness, primitive living, and group responsibility for many of the long-term therapeutic camps still in existence today, including Eckerd Youth

Alternatives (founded in 1968) in Florida, Pressley Ridge Ohiopyle (founded in 1975) in Pennsylvania, and Three Springs (founded in 1985) in Alabama, the most notorious of the long-term therapeutic camps, Anneewakee Treatment Center, (founded in 1962) in Georgia will be reviewed at the end of this chapter.

The majority of early therapeutic camps developed out of mental health organizations (referred to as "mental hygiene" in the early 1900's) or civic organizations that wanted to integrate camping and the outdoors into the treatment. Those organizations included the Jewish Board of Guardians, Massachusetts General Hospital, Dallas Salesmanship Club, and University of Michigan. The founders of many of the camps were mental health professionals including psychiatrists, social workers, and psychologists who staffed their camps with the like. Some camps that are still in existence today, including Ramapo for Children and Camp Wediko, continue to employ an extensive mental health professional staff. (These camps primarily operate during the summer months.)

The Dallas Salesmanship Club Camp, with its long-term focus, exclusion of mental health professionals, and wilderness trips with psychologically challenged youth, helped to usher in an entirely new era in the field. This era could be characterized by a movement away from mental health professionals and towards multi-day wilderness trips facilitated by people with strong outdoor skills. This type of process can also be attributed to Outward Bound, whose founder, Kurt Hahn, also had a strong distaste for mental health professionals.

1941: Outward Bound

The Outward Bound organization had a profound impact on the field of wilderness therapy. The founder of Outward Bound was Kurt Hahn who, giving credit to the ideas of others including Baden-Powell (founder of Boy Scouts) and Plato, developed much of the philosophy and theoretical foundation of the field of wilderness therapy and outdoor education. In *Kurt Hahn's School and Legacy,* an alumnus of the Salem School, Martin Flavin (1996) writes that Hahn was "born in 1886 into a cultivated Jewish family in Berlin, Germany, whose affluence stemmed from his paternal grandfather" (p. 2). Interestingly, Hahn suffered sunstroke so severe as a 19 year old that he had to avoid direct light and heat throughout his life. But this malady did not handicap his love of learning, nor greatly hinder his influence on peers! Hahn attended Oxford in 1910 where he made many friends and influential contacts while he studied philosophy of education with a distinct interest in Plato; as you'll read, these same contacts would be useful to him later in life when he was forced to leave an increasingly anti-Semitic Germany.

After World War I, Hahn became secretary to Prince Max von Baden, the last Imperial Chancellor of Germany, who financed Hahn's Salem School in 1920. It is there that Hahn wrote the Seven Laws of Salem in 1930, documenting what still could be overarching principles of modern wilderness therapy:

1. Give the children opportunities for self-discovery.

2. Make the children meet with triumph and defeat.

3. Give the children the opportunity of self-effacement in the common cause.

4. Provide periods of silence.

5. Train the imagination.

6. Make games important but not predominant.

7. Free the sons of the wealthy and powerful from the enervating sense of privilege. (Flavin, 1996, p. 15)

Hahn's laws related to "freeing the sons of the wealthy from the enervating sense of privilege" were similar to the philosophy of the Camp Chocorua Principles. Hahn emphasized that the goal of the school, similar to Boy Scouting, was "character training" (Flavin, 1996, p. 17). As Director, he divided the staff into two categories: teachers and character trainers. He believed strongly in educating the young in areas of character yet, similar to Loughmiller, he did not have high regard for mental health professionals. Hahn "is said to have taken charge aggressively in cases of serious illness: he would cause a doctor a great deal of woe if he felt any doubt about his ministrations, and knew where all the best specialists were to be found and how to get them interested – except for psychiatrists, whom he thoroughly distrusted" (Flavin, 1996, p. 117). Hahn's Salem School could be seen as one of the first character-based boarding school in the world, yet because his direction of Salem swirled amid the turmoil of pre-Nazi Germany, Hahn's allegiance to character cut short his new duty.

According to Flavin (1996), Hahn wrote a letter to the Salem School alumni and parents, in 1933, requiring them to make what he thought was a principled, ethical choice – to terminate either their relationship with Hitler and the Nazi movement or their relationship with the school, which of course infuriated the newly elected Nazi regime. Hahn was briefly jailed and, shortly thereafter, with the intervention of his Oxford colleagues, was exiled to Great Britain. There, with help from his influential friends, he conceived a whole series of new educational ventures including the Gordonstoun School and Outward Bound. Hahn requested and swore allegiance to Britain in 1938, and converted to the Church of England in 1945. If it were not for Hahn's disdain of Hitler and the Nazi regime, it can safely be assumed that Outward Bound may not have ever existed.

Josh Miner, founder of Outward Bound USA, and co-author Joe Boldt detail Hahn's emigration to Great Britain, the founding of Gordonstoun and eventually the Outward Bound programs, in *Outward Bound USA: Crew Not Passengers* (1981). When Hahn arrived in Great Britain, at the age of 47, he was profoundly depressed; "he had lost his homeland, his school, and the battle for German youth" (p. 34). When asked to start a school similar to Salem School, Hahn stated he "lacked the will" (p. 34). Months later, he found a location in an empty castle near the sea, and he opened the Gordonstoun School in 1934. Hahn would recall these lonely months as instrumental in bringing to him an insight that he would share with others: "Your disability is your opportunity" (p. 34). Five years later, as the Axis and Allied powers have declared war, the British Army commandeered the Gordonstoun School, and Hahn's school moved to a safer location in Wales. Coincidentally, "Hahn had been trying to launch a 'County Badge scheme' that fostered physical fitness, enterprise, tenacity, and compassion among British youth" (p. 35). The County Badge did not gain a large following until Lawrence Holt, a Gordonstoun School parent, Hahn admirer, and partner in a large shipping company, approached Hahn about the loss of life of young seaman in the Battle of the Atlantic. Holt wanted to develop a national program to train young people, especially sailors, to have "reliance on their own resources, and selfless bound with their fellows." Subsequently, Hahn and Holt joined forces to start a "new kind of school offering one-month courses that would use Hahn's County Badge scheme to implement Holt's quest for training to turn attitudes around" (p. 35). They named the program "Outward Bound," a nautical term for when a ship is leaving port to the open ocean. This was much to Hahn's dislike but chosen upon Holt's insistence and financial backing of the program. Outward Bound opened in 1941 in Aberdovey, Wales. The first Outward Bound program was a rigorous month-long course of small boat training, athletic experiences, map and compass skills, rescue training, an expedition at sea, and a land expedition across three mountain ranges, as well as service to local people. Thus began a movement that would not only influence youth in Britain, but all around the world. Despite Outward Bound's success, the theories and philosophies that drove the program were not well documented and can only be attributed to several speeches given by Hahn.

On July 20, 1960, two years before Outward Bound arrived in the United States, Kurt Hahn gave a lecture to the Outward Bound Trust that outlined the origins and philosophy behind Outward Bound. In the lecture, Hahn exhibited his humility and wit, while he pointed to several key historical influences to the evolution of Outward Bound. Those influences included the Boy Scouts, Plato, and public schools:

> "Do not regard me as the originator either of the diagnosis or the cure which I advocate. Perhaps I can best illustrate what I mean by telling you of a remark which my late Chief Prince Max of Baden once made when he was guiding an over-enthusiastic American through his school. The American said to the Prince, "Would you mind telling me what are you proudest of in these beautiful schools?" And Prince Max said, "If you go the length and breadth of them, there's nothing original in them. That is what I am proud of. We have stolen from everywhere, from the Boy Scouts, from Plato, from Goethe and from the public schools." And the American said: "Ought you not to aim at being original?" and Prince Max answered, "No, it is in education as in medicine. You must harvest the wisdom of a thousand years. If ever you come to a surgeon and he wants to take out your appendix in the most original manner possible, I would

strongly advise you to go to another surgeon." (Hahn, 1960)

Later in the address, Hahn described how Outward Bound addresses the challenges of youth:

"These four elements – fitness training, expeditions, projects, rescue service are familiar to all who have experienced or witnessed Outward Bound in action. I should like to call them antidotes. When you speak of an antidote, you imply that the human organism has to be protected against poison. There can be no doubt that the young of today have to be protected against certain poisonous effects inherent in present-day civilization." (Hahn, 1960)

He then expanded on what he saw as the "five social diseases" for the young in society:

"Five social diseases surround them, even in early childhood. There is the decline in fitness due to the modern methods of locomotion, the decline in initiative, due to the widespread disease of spectatoritis, the decline in care and skill, due to the weakened tradition of craftsmanship, the decline in self-discipline, due to the ever-present availability of tranquilizers and stimulants, the decline of compassion, which William Temple called "spiritual death." (Hahn, 1960)

The "social diseases" that Hahn discussed are not only as relevant today but they continue to increase, as technology and medical science improve.

Hahn also covered how to motivate the young in his talk:

"There are three ways of trying to win the young. There is persuasion, there is compulsion and there is attraction. You can preach at them, that is a hook without a worm; you can say "You must volunteer," that is of the devil; and you can tell them, "You are needed." That appeal hardly ever fails. I am quite certain that the young of today respond better to the service which is demanded from them in the interest of others than to the service which is offered them for their overt benefit and improvement." (Hahn, 1960)

Hahn's focus on service to others and the encouragement of youth through a message of "you are needed" comes from Hahn's belief in the fable of the Good Samaritan. "I believe that the challenge of Samaritan Service, if properly presented, rarely fails to capture young people, body and soul, not only in the Western World" (Miner, Boldt, & Eno, 1981, p. 350). This outward focus is summarized in Outward Bound's motto, appropriated from Alfred, Lord Tennyson's poem *Ulysses*"... to serve, to strive, and not to yield." Before his death in 1974, Hahn was able to see Outward Bound USA begin the transformative era of wilderness therapy, which will be chronicled in the next chapter. Yet before ending this chapter, it is important to identify and review the most controversial long-term therapeutic camp, Anneewakee, which was founded in 1962.

1962: Anneewakee

Anneewakee, a Cherokee name for "land of the friendly people," was founded, directed, and owned by Louis "Doc" Poetter, (who held neither a medical license nor a doctorate degree) in 1962 in Georgia (Corvette, 1986). The model was a long-term therapeutic wilderness camp, similar to the Salesmanship Club Camp, in which youths would construct campsites and live for up to sixteen months. The campsites were dotted throughout the property where there was also a main eating facility and administrative buildings. Unlike the Salesmanship Club Camp, the program was staffed with mental health professionals. The program would expand to have two camps, one for girls in Georgia and one for boys in Florida.

In a series of reports in *The Atlanta Journal* by David Corvette, the abusive culture of Anneewakee was fully exposed and chronicled. Corvette wrote in 1986 that after "two months of intense investigation at Anneewakee, an expensive, non-profit hospital that stresses wilderness therapy for troubled youths, the Douglas County Sheriff's Department and the Georgia Bureau of Investigation filed charges against Anneewakee employees [including Poetter]" (p. D1). These were not the first sexual abuse charges against Poetter as "rumors of abuse have whirled around Anneewakee at least since 1970, when a former therapist accused Poetter in a lawsuit of having sexual relations with patients" (p. D1). The plea deal after the 1970 charges was that Anneewakee kept its license as a treatment program and Poetter would keep his executive director job, but was not allowed to visit youths at the camp.

Corvette (1990) would later report, in a follow up article on the criminal investigation of Anneewakee, that Poetter pled guilty to nineteen counts of sodomy of patients and was sentenced to eight years in prison. Other Anneewakee staff would also be charged and found guilty of sexual abuse. The Anneewakee facility would be found guilty of fraud as they overbilled insurance companies and families for treatment provided by psychologists. Former clients would sue and win a successful lawsuit against Anneewakee claiming they were forced to build and repair the facilities and were cheated out of the education and therapy for which their parents had paid. In 1987, Annewakkee would be forced by the Georgia Department of Human Resources to be given over to the Hospital Corporation of America who would manage the day-to-day operations.

Anneewakee is the most controversial long-term wilderness therapy camp identified in this section. Although it started in 1962, its long-term camp model can be traced to the Dallas Salesmanship Club Camp. Anneewakee is included in this chapter for it emerged from the camp model and is the earliest example of a long-term program to conceal vast abuse and financial improprieties behind the banner of therapy. Unfortunately, others will be revealed in the next chapter.

Summary

This chapter identified the early organizations that helped shape what would become wilderness therapy. It chronicles a movement from character training in summer camps (Camp Chocorua) and outdoor programs (Boy Scouting) to summer camps for "problem children" (Camp Ramapo) to long term youth camps (Salesmanship Club Camp). As earlier mentioned, the first multi-day wilderness expeditions with troubled youth in the United States occurred at the Salesmanship Club Camp. Although never explicitly stated as "therapy" by Kurt Hahn, Outward Bound appears to have been developed to be an "antidote" to the "social diseases" of modern youth. Many of these early organizations were practicing what would now be referred to as "wilderness therapy."

Regardless of the representation, these early organizations are the foundation of the wilderness therapy field and set the stage for the explosion of wilderness therapy programs for youth in the latter half of the twentieth century.

Chapter 2

1962-2012: Transformation from Wilderness Survival to Wilderness Therapy to Outdoor Behavioral Healthcare

THE PERIOD FROM 1962 TO 2012 MARKS A major transformation in the field of wilderness therapy. Many of the early organizations of this period focused on either primitive skills or mountaineering styles of expeditions as an avenue for change for young people. During the 1960s, two vastly different organizations would open their doors to American teenagers and young adults – Outward Bound USA and Brigham Young University's "BYU 480 Class: Youth Rehabilitation through Outdoor Survival." These two organizations would lead to a profound acceleration of the use of outdoor experiences to help change the character of youth. The majority of wilderness therapy programs in existence today can be traced to one of these two organizations, or to the Dallas Salesmanship Club Camp of Dallas.

The 1970's were the inception of some of the first outdoor-based organizations to work with adjudicated youth (Becket Academy, Outward Bound, Expedition Outreach, VisionQuest), public school programs (Project Adventure), and mental health organizations (Outward Bound Mental Health Project). In this same decade, the first documents using the term "wilderness therapy" would emerge, as well as the first organization for practitioners of the field, the Association for Experiential Education (AEE).

It was during the 1980's that numerous organizations would open in the west (Wilderness Treatment Center, School of Urban and Wilderness Survival, Anasazi Foundation, Aspen Achievement Academy, Wilderness

Quest, Catherine Freer Wilderness), many of which were for-profit and based on the primitive survival skills expedition model first practiced at BYU 480. The 1980's are also when another notorious wilderness therapy organization, the Challenger Foundation, opened its doors. This organization, and similarly styled programs later started by some of its former employees, was one of several documented organizations that created climates of intimidation and disrespect that led to the deaths of several youths.

In the 1990's and beyond, wilderness therapy caught the public eye, and a variety of books, articles, and a television series made it into the mainstream. Simultaneously, several professional organizations were formed, in direct reaction to the independent and unobserved nature of the recent abuses. In the last ten years, a call for greater regulation by government officials has occurred. In addition, there has been a movement to adopt a new term for the field of wilderness therapy and a push for more research into the effectiveness of this therapeutic approach. The beginning of this section starts with Outward Bound USA, which is arguably the most influential organization in the development of wilderness therapy, due to its broad impact on the field.

1962: Outward Bound USA

According to Miner, Boldt and Eno (1981), Outward Bound was brought to the United States by Josh Miner. Miner, after serving in World War II and then graduating from Princeton University, worked at The Hun School in Princeton, New Jersey. In 1950, Miner was approached by his father-in-law, Jack Stevens, a successful businessman who was involved with international business and politics. Stevens had been asked to "help raise money for the work being done by a German headmaster of a school in Scotland" (p. 17). Stevens told Miner of this Gordonstoun School in Scotland and its German headmaster, Kurt Hahn, who was also involved with "some-kind of outdoor and rescue training school" that many believed could be a "helpful influence on postwar Germany" (p. 18). Stevens asked Miner to go spend some time with Hahn and write a report about it. Miner went to Scotland and studied what Hahn was involved with and wrote the report. Miner was so impressed that he returned, in 1951, with his whole family to be faculty at Gordonstoun and to work directly with Hahn. Miner was whole-heartedly inspired by the "outdoor and rescue training school," which was now formally named Outward Bound, and brought the concept to the United States.

The first American school, Colorado Outward Bound, opened on June 16, 1962. The 26-day course started at a base camp in the Rocky Mountains where participants were trained in needed skills such as map and compass, backpacking, first aid, knots, rock climbing, firefighting and mountain rescue followed by several multi-day expeditions. The first course also included a six-mile run, a "marathon" in OB argot, at the end of the course and a single "night alone." During the second course in the school's fledgling program, the cook informed the chief instructor, "Tap" Tapley, that their food supplier would not arrive for several days due to difficulties on the mountain roads. Tapley gathered the staff around and told them, "Tonight we'll get the group together, and I'll give them a talk on edible plants and berries, and what kinds of game and fish they can find to eat, and we'll tell them they're going on a three-day solo survival" (Miner et al., 1981, p. 109). Thus, due to a lack of food supply for students during the second Outward Bound USA course, the tradition of three days by oneself in the wild, termed a "solo," first started in the US. The "solo" and the practice of completing a final "marathon" run are now long-standing traditions in Outward Bound courses as well as many wilderness therapy programs.

Colorado Outward Bound had a variety of challenges to start out with, including that its founder, Josh Miner, similar to Hahn, was an expert at motivating young people but had limited outdoor skills. What Miner did have was a passion for Outward Bound, and he went about hiring some of the most famous mountaineers at the time. Colorado Outward Bound became a magnet for mountaineers who were attracted to the organization and its flexible work schedule, which supported extended time off for climbing expeditions. These mountaineers would influence the organization by insisting that high-quality tents, sleeping bags, and climbing gear be integrated into the model. The most famous for his legendary climbs was the opinionated mountaineer, Paul Petzoldt who became the chief instructor of Colorado Outward Bound in 1963 (Ringholz, 1998). Petzoldt soon became disenchanted with Outward Bound, as he felt instructors were poorly trained: "I practically told them their school was never going to amount to a goddamn unless they had an instructor's training program" (Ringholz, 1998, p. 180). Petzoldt would leave Outward Bound USA and start his own training programs called the National Outdoor Leadership School, in 1965, and the Wilderness Education Association, in 1977 (Ringholz, 1998, p.180). Petzoldt's criticism about lack of staff training would later haunt the organization. Yet he was wrong about the organization never amounting to anything. Outward Bound USA would spread like a wildfire in the 1960s and influence many individuals who, like Petzoldt, would start other organizations.

Outward Bound expanded rapidly in the US throughout the 1960s by opening six schools, in Colorado, Maine, Minnesota, Oregon, North Carolina, and New Hampshire. In 1965, the gender barrier was broken in the U.S. by Bob Pieh, head of Minnesota Outward Bound, who offered the first girls' course (Miner et al., 1981). While Outward Bound was expanding in the U.S., it maintained an association with private boarding schools through Miner's position as a faculty member at the prestigious Philips Academy in Andover, MA. Hahn and Miner had always been involved in independent schools, and many of their Outward Bound USA instructors worked at boarding schools during the academic year. Miner was concerned that the "movement would acquire a 'preppie' stigma" and would only be available to the teens with wealthy parents (Miner et al., 1981, p. 38). To combat this, they started a policy that one-half of an Outward Bound USA school's enrollments should be given scholarships. Miner went about implementing this policy by developing programs for adjudicated and troubled youth. To put it simply, Outward Bound USA began working with adjudicated youth to avoid being seen as just a program for rich, prep school kids.

1966: Outward Bound for Adjudicated Youth

In the summer of 1966, several Outward Bound USA schools around the country enrolled sixty adjudicated youth who were under the custody of the Massachusetts Department of Youth Services. The enrollment of these sixty youth was to see if the experience would lead to less recidivism when compared to a control group of adjudicated delinquent youth who did not attend Outward Bound USA (Kelly & Baer, 1968). This was the first of numerous research studies looking at the effectiveness of Outward Bound USA on reducing recidivism in adjudicated, delinquent youth. The experiment was a relative success with twenty percent of the Outward

Bound USA group reoffending compared to thirty-seven percent of the control group (Kelly & Baer, 1968). The research outcome caused a surge in requests for Outward Bound to provide more courses for adjudicated youth. Outward Bound began to offer courses all over the country to serve this population.

1975: Outward Bound for Mentally Ill Adolescents and Adults

The first documented integration of Outward Bound for mentally ill adolescents and adults occurred in 1975 in association with Dartmouth-Hitchcock Mental Health Center in Hanover, New Hampshire (Stich, 1983). In an article titled "Experiential Therapy," Thomas Stich, who was the director of the Outward Bound Mental Health Project, described the program as collaboration between Dartmouth Medical School and Hurricane Island Outward Bound. The organization served as an outpatient, an inpatient, and a residential treatment program. "The purpose of the Dartmouth Outward Bound Mental Health Project is to develop a unique, patient education program that utilizes not only traditional concepts of patient education but also experiential learning" (Stich, 1983, p.30). The program did not take participants on overnight trips but had six to eight hour experiences, including cross-country skiing, canoeing, and rock climbing. The program closed in the 1980s.

1983: Outward Bound for Inpatient Adolescent Substance Abuse Treatment

The first documented integration of the Outward Bound Program and inpatient adolescent substance abuse treatment occurred at Beech Hill Hospital located in Dublin, New Hampshire, starting in 1983. McPeake, Kennedy, Grossman, and Beaulieu (1991), who were all staff in the program, reviewed this model in an article titled "Innovative Adolescent Chemical Dependency Treatment and Its Outcome: A Model Based on Outward Bound Programming." This program was two-part; the three-day assessment phase occurring at the hospital, which helped to develop the treatment plan, and the twenty-two-day wilderness phase, facilitated by Outward Bound-certified instructors and Master's level clinical staff, in which participants would hike or canoe in the New Hampshire or Maine Wilderness and culminate in a 48-hour solo. This unique program was short-lived. It closed in the early 1990s followed by Beech Hill Hospital closing in 2001.

It is well documented (Godfrey, 1980; Miner et al., 1981; Ringholz, 1998) that those involved in the early days of Outward Bound USA went on to start many of the most prominent outdoor organizations today, including National Outdoor Leadership School (NOLS), Wilderness Education Association (WEA), Project Adventure and countless other programs and associations in the United States. Outward Bound is globally recognized as at the vanguard of outdoor education.

Despite its success, the Outward Bound USA organization has also had its share of controversies, including a well-publicized death that highlights some of the differences between a licensed wilderness therapy program and a wilderness program for "normal" adolescents.

Controversy at Outward Bound

In a May 2007 article, titled "A Death at Outward Bound," journalist Christopher Ketcham examined the circumstances surrounding the July 2006 heat stroke death of an Outward Bound student, Elisa, during a Utah desert expedition.

"Elisa was the first Outward Bound student to die in almost a decade and the 24th fatality in the nonprofit's 46-year history in the U.S." (Ketcham, 2007, p. 49) Ketchum revealed that most of the twenty-four deaths at Outward Bound USA happened prior to the 1980s. In this most recent death, Ketcham notes that the organization's response was a deafening silence to the specifics of the case. A small group of insiders spoke out and warned that Outward Bound's safety standards had fallen "disturbingly low" (Ketcham, 2007, p. 49). The article describe the views of some former Outward Bound instructors who believed the organization was not training its new instructors in basic wilderness medicine, behavioral de-escalation, group management skills, as well as not retaining older, more seasoned staff.

Despite a good safety record over the years, this criticism of poor staff training at Outward Bound, first brought up by Paul Petzoldt, caused internal changes attending to instructor competence at Outward Bound. In December of 2006, the President of Outward Bound USA, Arthur

Blank (cofounder of Home Depot), donated over one million dollars to the organization for increased professional training for instructors.

Interestingly, many wilderness therapy programs were taking place in the same area as the Outward Bound course in which Elisa died but, because of State of Utah wilderness therapy program licensure regulations, they were prohibited from hiking if the temperature was over 90 degrees (Ketcham, 2007, p. 54). The Outward Bound course that Elisa attended was not listed as therapeutic, so it did not have to follow Utah therapeutic licensure regulations. Sadly, the day after Elisa died, an adult participant in the Boulder Outdoor Survival School, which also was not required to follow licensing standards, died in Utah from dehydration.

This same media attention would later be directed at therapeutic camps and wilderness therapy programs.

Significance of Outward Bound on Wilderness Therapy

Outward Bound USA's significance in the evolution of wilderness therapy cannot be overstated. It created a movement that, through its numerous locations, exposed many people, and the nation, to the idea of personal growth through challenging adventure. Outward Bound is a critical organization as its mountaineering expeditionary model – with staged increases in responsibility and independence, following displayed group competence – has been replicated or modified by many in the wilderness therapy field. Kurt Hahn's theories of working with youth continue to be seen in wilderness therapy programs as well as character-based educational organizations. Outward Bound would inspire many advocates through their direct experiences with the program and a select few would subsequently modify the Outward Bound curriculum to start new organizations. Some of the early wilderness therapy organizations inspired by the Outward Bound model, or started with former Outward Bound staff, include Penikese Island School in Massachusetts (founded in 1973 and closed in 2010), Wilderness School in Connecticut (founded in 1974), and Blackwater Outdoor Experiences in Virginia (founded in 1980). One organization that evolved simultaneously and separately from Outward Bound was Becket Academy. Becket Academy would start numerous wilderness therapy programs as well as hold the first conference dedicated solely to wilderness therapy.

1964: Becket Academy

Founded by Dr. John Wolter, with the help of his wife, Joan Wolter, the school opened its doors in 1964 in East Haddam, Connecticut. Later Becket Academy would expand its operations with additional schools and programs in New Hampshire and Florida. The Wolters and their teams would develop numerous wilderness therapy programs for different populations, up and down the East Coast. What is interesting about Becket Academy and the Wolters is that many of their progressive ideas in the 1960s and 1970s, such as incorporating yoga, organic foods, and meditation, as well as challenging wilderness expeditions, are, once again, in the forefront of the field. It is additionally remarkable that their organization founded the first conference dedicated solely to the field of wilderness therapy. Becket Academy's story is well documented in a doctoral dissertation, by Doug Teschner, titled "A Case Study in Educational Innovation: Becket Academy 1964-1984" (1985).

In 1977, and due to changes in the State of Connecticut special education funding, Becket Academy would transition from working with a traditional population to become an accredited schools for behaviorally challenged young people. By 1981, every student placed at these schools was funded by public agencies (Teschner, 1985, p. 315).

Along with these changes to the student body, Becket Academy started to develop outdoor programs in New Hampshire for students who were not doing well at the Connecticut campus. The "Ranger Program" integrated outdoor activities, including hiking, backpacking, Nordic skiing and wilderness survival, as a month-long intervention for Becket Academy students (p. 260). During this period, Becket Academy developed a satellite campus in New Hampshire and continued to develop programs that were "a hybrid of applied academics (including field trips), farming and other work projects, wilderness expeditions, Marine Corp influences [Wolter was a veteran of the Marine Corps], endurance activities, and adventure/challenge program" (p. 272).

The Voyager program began in the winter of 1980 as a program for Becket Academy students "who had low sense of self-regard, refuse to adhere to limits, disregard instructions, and deny personal responsibility for the events and quality of their lives" (p. 303). The program integrated meditation, yoga, nutrition education, and substance abuse education into a longer term canoe and hiking expeditions (Voyager program manual). For over a month, staff and students would travel around to bases in the Everglades, Canada, and New Mexico where they would participate in outdoor activities until the students were deemed ready to return to Becket Academy's main campus. The Voyager program was relatively successful which inspired the Wolters and their team to develop Ultra, based on an island in the Everglades but travelling by van as far as Canada (p. 321).

Ultra worked primarily with troubled young people who were referred and paid for by their sending state, including Connecticut, Massachusetts, Vermont, and New Hampshire. The program was designed specifically for students who were not behaviorally capable of enrolling at Becket Academy, so they enrolled directly into Ultra. The program was abandoned, after several years, due to a 1982 incident in Canada in which Becket Academy's Ultra program staff were arrested at their camp site by Canadian officials. They were charged with child abuse, as well as working in the country without permits, and the students were placed in a Canadian detention facility. After many meetings between United States government officials, Becket Academy administration, and Canadian officials, the staff and students returned to the United States. Canadian officials did not bring charges of abuse, but they did press charges against the staff for working without a permit. The State of Connecticut would clear Becket Academy's Ultra staff of any wrongdoing. Negative press about the international conflict with Ultra caused Connecticut officials to become reluctant to send children to this program and Ultra was eventually shut down. Resulting news reports, developing difficulty with State of Connecticut contracts and John Wolter's frustration with bureaucracy would slowly have its impact on Becket Academy. Wolter would close the Becket Academy and Founders School in Connecticut and move to the Becket Academy New Hampshire campus, rebranding his program as the Pike School.

But before Becket Academy left Connecticut, the Wolters would start the Institute for Experiential Education, which founded the first conference dedicated solely to wilderness therapy. The Institute for Experiential Education (IEE) was founded on the idea that there needed to be "trained leaders to meet the growing demand of public and private organizations for professionals to work with persons having special needs" and would become focused primarily on those professionals working with youth in the out-of-doors (p. 327-328). Though short lived, the IEE held two conferences, in the spring of 1983 and 1984, for practitioners of what is now referred to as wilderness therapy. The first conference featured Bob Burton from VisionQuest and Dr. Richard Kimball from the Santa Fe Mountain Center (both programs will be profiled in this section) and was featured in a newspaper article titled "Wilderness Conference to Explore Youth Programs" (*The Gazette*, May 19, 1983, page 8). The second conference, in April of 1984, featured Josh Miner from Outward Bound and Campbell Loughmiller from the Dallas Salesmanship Club Camp (both programs profiled already in this book). There are neither records of a third conference nor indications of why the Institute of Experiential Education closed.

Becket Academy would be the first to adopt longer wilderness expeditions in a boarding school for behaviorally challenged youth. They would create numerous programs, some documented and others not, that would incorporate wilderness therapy practices as an intervention for youth. Dr. John Wolter would pass away in 2004, but his legacy for creating numerous innovative schools and programs for youth would continue through his son, Jay Wolter, who has served as President of what is now known as the "Becket Family of Services" since 1993. Under Jay's leadership, Becket Academy has grown to encompass numerous sites throughout New England that primarily serve youth and young adults with very significant behavioral disorders. These programs remain holistically focused, but have greatly de-emphasized wilderness therapy as a primary treatment modality. Becket Academy has also played an important role in the founding of several recent ventures that are influenced by the Wolter legacy, including the independently operated Oliverian School and the Mountain Valley Treatment Center.

1968: Brigham Young University 480: Youth Rehabilitation through Outdoor Survival

Of the thousands of participants who were motivated and moved by Outward Bound experiences, one particularly accomplished Instructor's experience with Colorado Outward Bound would spark a movement in the West that would bring the integration of primitive survival skills into wilderness therapy. With Larry Dean Olsen's attempt to give some failing students a second chance at college by creating Brigham Young University's "480 Class: Youth Rehabilitation through Outdoor Survival," Olsen initiated what would become the dispersion of wilderness therapy programs, wilderness-oriented weekends at residential treatment facilities and even state governmental support for the explosion of programming in Utah.

In 1967, Larry Dean Olsen graduated from Brigham Young University (BYU) with a degree in elementary education, and in conjunction with his school work, published a book titled *Outdoor Survival Skills*. With these two life experiences, Olsen became renowned as one of the country's leading experts in the area of primitive survival skills and their potential use in wilderness programs. In that summer, Olsen was invited by the Colorado Outward Bound School to teach their staff about survival skills, but when he arrived, Outward Bound was short-staffed so they hired him to work on a couple of courses. Olsen had been taking people out on survival trips for ten days at a time while Outward Bound trips were typically 28 days. After helping Outward Bound, Olsen recognized that he could safely take students out for longer periods of time and incorporate some of the Outward Bound practices, such as solos and a final run, into primitive skills survival trips.

In 1968, the Academic Standards Committee at BYU asked Olsen to build a program and then supervise 26 students who had failed out of BYU the previous semester, on a month-long primitive skills class. This first class was referred to by students as "BYU 480," which was the course number for the class, and its purpose was to give failing students an opportunity for readmission to BYU. BYU 480 was a challenging program. It included a day of training in primitive survival skills followed by a twenty-eight-day desert expedition equipped with the clothes the students were wearing, a knife, a sleeping bag, a canteen of water, and a small amount of food. During the first course, a student named Ezekiel Sanchez helped Olsen when the only other leader on the trip dropped out after two days. Sanchez would become instrumental to the teaching and implementation of BYU 480 and other outdoor survival courses, as well as the development of wilderness therapy.

The first BYU 480 program was deemed a success, leading to Olsen and Sanchez' course and vision becoming critical to the development of BYU's Youth Leadership Department. BYU began to offer the primitive skills expedition courses to anyone who wanted to learn primitive survival skills while also providing other classes and seminars to learn primitive survival skills. Students of these survival courses were experiencing profound individual changes. The word of this spread from BYU through the Church of Jesus Christ of Latter Day Saints (LDS) community as, according to the BYU website, 98% of students are LDS. A number of individuals who took the class would subsequently start primitive skills wilderness survival programs for adolescents. The BYU Survival Programs swelled with scout leaders, probation officers, and others interested in promoting character development in youth. Olsen, Sanchez, and BYU 480 would be seen as catalysts for many of the wilderness therapy programs that emerged in the West that use primitive survival skills as a therapeutic tool in working with troubled adolescents. Olsen would later be credited with inspiring the founding of the Boulder Outdoor Survival School (BOSS) in the late 1960s, which is the first primitive skills survival training organization for adults (Boulder Outdoor Survival School website, 2011). Olsen and Sanchez would both leave BYU in the 1970s in order to pursue other interests, but would collaborate again in 1988 to start the Anasazi Foundation (see Section 2 of this book).

After Olsen and Sanchez left BYU 480, a research project examined the outline and effects of the course on participants. The psychological and sociological effects on students of BYU 480 were the subject of a 1976 doctoral dissertation by Kenneth Seymour. Seymour (1976) described the course, at that time, as having five phases:

1. **Impact** – Each student becomes adjusted to the environment through three days of rigorous hiking.

2. **Group Expedition** – Men and women are put in separate groups; each group, with instructor assistance, follows a prescribed route to a common destination.

3. **Survival week** – focused on using primitive outdoor survival

skills.

4. **Student Expedition** – Students are organized into small groups and given specifics to follow to a common destination.

5. **Solo** – Each student spends from four to five days alone in a selected supervised area

This challenging course would last 28 days and occur in southern Utah where students would hike 250 miles of alpine and desert terrain.

Seymour (1976) reviewed some of the psychological impacts of the class, as students "see more clearly their reason for existing and find life more meaningful. They see a mission or a purpose in life. A significant number discovered more clear cut goals, and in general, find life over all more satisfying after Outdoor Survival" (p. 70). Although the subjects in this research included many members of the LDS faith, there were also participants who were not LDS. According to Seymour, "A BYU 28 day wilderness experience creates conflict among those not of the LDS faith" (p. 70). Seymour found that several non-LDS participants converted to the LDS faith while on the course and when they returned home they were not supported by family who were not LDS.

This study also documented a death during the second day of this researched course: "A 24 year old female was stricken while on a forced march, identified as 'Impact', and died of dehydration before help could be summoned" (Seymour, 1976, p. 490). Seymour's dissertation is the only document uncovered by this author focused on the psychological impact of the BYU 480 course and is the only document to cite the death of a participant in BYU 480. After the death of the student at BYU 480, the course would become available only to Outdoor Recreation majors and then was subsequently phased out by BYU in the early 1980s. The Boulder Outdoor Survival School (BOSS) would later provide a similar experience as the BYU 480 model, but in the private sector.

1971: Expedition Outreach and Larry Wells

The first primitive skills based wilderness therapy expeditions for adjudicated youth started in 1971, in Challis, Idaho, at a program named Expedition Outreach, founded by BYU 480 alumnus Larry Wells. Stephen Watts (2003), a former Idaho state investigator, wrote a book titled *Better an Honest Scoundrel: Chronicle of a Western Lawman*, which identified Expedition Outreach as a private non-profit program to help struggling young people via primitive survival expeditions, with Larry Wells as the first executive director. Watts first became acquainted with Wells in the 1960s after he arrested him for assault with a deadly weapon. Watts kept track of Wells during his time in prison and subsequent rehabilitation. Watts was so impressed with Wells' rehabilitation that he successfully petitioned the Governor of Idaho for a pardon for Wells.

After release, Wells went to work for the United States Forest Service and then attended a BYU 480 instructor's class (Watts, 2003, p. 121). After completing the BYU 480 instructor class, Wells approached Watts and Darroll Gardiner, a probation officer, to develop a program for adjudicated youth. They all worked together to start a non-profit organization named Expedition Outreach. Like the BYU 480 course, Expedition Outreach's goals were to provide supervised but challenging extended experiences to members of a peer group, supported by individual primitive survival skills training and general teamwork skills-practice. An Expedition Outreach course lasted 30 days in which a mixed population of (adjudicated and "regular population") students were "marched into the wilderness areas and taught to live off the land, fend for themselves, and rely on partnerships with others to survive" (Watts, 2003, p. 121). This organization was open to people over the age of fifteen and included adjudicated participants, some of whom were referred from Idaho State Prison, the State Reformatory, and individuals on probation, as well as non-adjudicated participants. The organization combined adults and adolescents into one group for these trips.

1973: VisionQuest

One of the largest, most successful organizations Wells would assist in starting was named VisionQuest. VisionQuest was formed in 1973 as one of the first private for-profit organizations that integrated the outdoors for rehabilitation of adjudicated and behaviorally challenged youth. This was a departure from previous adjudicated programs developed by Outward Bound and others, which were primarily not-for-profit programs. In his book *A Path with Honor: The Story of VisionQuest,* Dennis Adams (1987), a former superior court judge who referred youth to the program, illuminates the history of VisionQuest. Bob Burton, a former corrections worker, founded the program because he was tired of the lack of innovation in the field and saw little success with the way state-run corrections facilities were working with youth. Burton, who had been a volunteer with the Crow Nation, felt that First Nation People rituals would benefit adjudicated youth. Burton established VisionQuest as a for-profit as he wanted the stockholders to be his employees who would also control the company. Burton approached Phoenix Youth Corrections and proposed a pilot project in which he would take adolescents out of "lock up" for a seven-day mountain expedition without charge. The Phoenix Youth Corrections program agreed to Burton's offer and, with the help of Larry Wells, the first VisionQuest expedition set out on a hundred-mile journey. Wells taught the students basic survival skills, map and compass skills, how to eat snakes and other gathered edibles, and how to rappel down cliffs. The trip was a difficult one, but the youth came back beaming and expressing their newfound insights to their corrections officers. Shortly thereafter, VisionQuest received $36,000 from the State of Arizona for special juvenile justice projects. This first trip provided credibility and enough cash to grow and add others to its start-up team.

Burton and VisionQuest's start-up team included Dr. Herbert Lazarus, a psychiatrist and author of a book entitled, *How to Get Your Money's Worth Out of Psychiatry*. Lazarus believed psychiatry was not helping anyone and that most outpatient mental health professionals were "just out to make a buck" (Adams, 1987, p. 120). Lazarus respected VisionQuest's treatment focus, in that it was action-oriented (Adams, 1987, p. 120). VisionQuest expanded quickly, adding group homes and other innovative outdoor programs for adjudicated youth across the nation, including supporting staff and students in horse driven wagon trains in which they would cross the country, as well as groups aboard sailing ships that would travel up and down the coast, referred to as OceanQuest.

In 1974, VisionQuest obtained approval from the Joint Commission on Accreditation of Hospitals, making it the first outdoor program to become accredited by this national organization. This allowed VisionQuest to seek insurance reimbursement for behaviorally challenged adolescents, as Burton was intent on not relying solely on State-run contracts. During the 1970s, VisionQuest grew by expanding beyond Arizona to other states, including Colorado and New Mexico. VisionQuest's influence on the field of wilderness therapy can be seen in several ways, including being one of the first programs to be Joint Commission accredited, being one of the first for-profit organizations, and for its different approaches (e.g., wagon trains, tall ships).

VisonQuest became involved in controversy in the 1970s with its regular use of confrontation with teens. In 1978, the Arizona Department of Economic Security had received 127 allegations of wrongdoing related to VisionQuest. They undertook a twelve-month investigation that, contrary to these allegations, ended with VisionQuest being reconfirmed with its licensure by the State of Arizona (Adams, 1987, p. 181-185). A 1988 report by the television news program *60 Minutes* again focused concern on the VisionQuest program (Eisen, 1988). In the exposé, news journalist Diane Sawyer stated, "dozens of people, present and former staff members included, told us that the majority of the staff who actually spend time with kids comes to the program with virtually no training and no experience in handling kids, much less severely delinquent ones." Sawyer confronted Bob Burton about the lack of training and low pay. Burton stated, "The entry staff is paid at the lowest that I could possibly pay them because I want to find out whether they can do this or not. Half the people that I hire cannot even do this job." Later on Burton stated, "no college is teaching anybody how to do this." Insufficient staff training and skills were not the only complaints in the report.

Sawyer interviewed Burt Johnson of the San Diego probation office, which had referred 390 juveniles to the VisionQuest program. Johnson stated, "I think that VisionQuest does not do what they purport to be able to do. I think they have an unqualified staff, they take unnecessary risk with children, they manipulate finances, and in general I feel they're irresponsible." Sawyer cited a study of the first 100 adjudicated boys sent to VisionQuest by San Diego probation. This study revealed that 92 percent were rearrested after discharge from the program.

VisionQuest was identified in 1995 as having 16 deaths associated with the program, some of which were staff (Krakauer, 1995). Nine of the deaths occurred in one sailing accident in November of 1980. According to the *60 Minutes* report, the United States Coast Guard did not cite VisionQuest for negligence in the sailing accident, but did say the vessel was not inspected, had too many people, and was run by an inexperienced crew (Eisen, 1998). Some of the criticisms leveled at VisionQuest (poor staff training, low wages) would be directed at the wilderness therapy field in general in the 2007 GAO investigation (see pg. 68).

VisionQuest currently operates in six states and provides services for adjudicated youth as well as non-adjudicated behaviorally challenged youth. Many individuals who worked for VisionQuest in the early years went on to be employed in other programs or started wilderness therapy programs on their own. During the same time that VisionQuest was opening its doors with a focus on treatment for adjudicated delinquent youth, a small organization named Project Adventure opened in the Northeast. This organization started what would later be referred to as adventure-based counseling and brought adventure therapy into schools and hospitals.

1971: Project Adventure and Adventure Based Counseling

According to Schoel, Prouty, and Radcliffe (1988), the explicit use of adventure for counseling purposes began at Project Adventure, founded in 1971 in Massachusetts by Jerry Pieh. Pieh was a former Outward Bound instructor and son of Bob Pieh, the founder of Minnesota Outward Bound. The aforementioned authors, all staff at Project Adventure, explained that Pieh felt that most young people could not afford the duration – as well as the physical and emotional cost – of a full Outward Bound course. Because of this, Pieh wanted to take the strategies used to develop the Outward Bound curriculum and adapt them for a traditional school setting. Although Project Adventure's focus was on all student populations, it soon developed as an alternative form of curriculum for at-risk students called "Adventure Based Counseling."

Two papers formed the foundation of *Adventure Based Counseling:* "Counseling on the Run" by Jim Schoel (1974) and "Confronting Passive Behavior through Outdoor Experience" by Rick Medrick (1979). Schoels (1974) wrote that, "Counseling on the run is a counseling relationship which provides growth through action" and a way of "connecting" with a student (p. 68). These articles were intended for anyone who worked with young people, including coaches, teachers, and counselors. Medrick's (1979) paper included the use of the outdoors, but also included the need for contracting and goal setting in order to systematize change for participants. Today, Adventure Based Counseling and related endeavors are generally referred to as "adventure therapy."

Schoel et al. (1988) revealed that Adventure Based Counseling was first practiced in 1974 by a mental health program at the Addison Gilbert Hospital and in a public high school course called the Action Seminar at Hamilton-Wenham Regional. The success of Adventure Based Counseling sparked a movement of integrating experiential activities into outpatient and inpatient treatment programs in order to create change. This movement was accelerated by Project Adventure's decision to publish a book on how to practice Adventure Based Counseling.

In 1988, Schoel et al. published *Islands of Healing: A Guide to Adventure Based Counseling*. They explained that the term "Islands of Healing" came from Kurt Hahn and that Project Adventure's plan was to become "small Outward Bound 'outposts' near major cities and international borders" (p. 4). As previously mentioned, Project Adventure recognized that many young people and their families could not afford the time or expense of a multi-day Outward Bound program; and so the idea was to bring an Outward Bound-type experience into schools and programs as "Adventure Based Counseling." They defined "Adventure Based Counseling as a dynamic, adaptive process" (p. xii) that quickly developed an ardent following. "Since the first Adventure Based Counseling workshop in May of 1979, over 2000 counselors, special needs teachers or therapist have been trained. Residential treatment centers, substance abuse clinics, state and county youth rehabilitation programs, school special needs departments and psychiatric hospitals have all turned to Project Adventure. Because of this trend the need for a text to help others think about and plan an effective Adventure Based Counseling adoption became increasingly obvious" (p. 8). *Islands of Healing: A Guide to Adventure Based Counseling* is the first publication to be focused on experiential activities as a process for change. The critical difference between adventure therapy and wilderness therapy is adventure therapy activities can occur in the indoors and outdoors, while wilderness therapy activities always take place in the outdoors over several days.

In 2002, an update of the book *Islands of Healing* was written by Jim Schoel and Richard Maizell and entitled *Exploring the Islands of Healing: New Perspectives on Adventure Based Counseling*. In this second edition, Schoel and Maizell changed course on Adventure Based Counseling's accessibility. In this printing, they explained that the "idea of Adventure Based Counseling (or Adventure Therapy, Experiential Therapy, etc.) has far outgrown the bailiwick of Project Adventure" (p. 10). They warned that the book "is not a substitute for training, education, or experience nor will reading it certify or license you to do anything" (p. xii). This is in stark contrast to *Islands of Healing* in which the authors state that the book allows the readers to understand Adventure Based Counseling so "that they can adapt, modify, and implement these ideas within their particular and unique workplaces" (p. xii). This updated book includes a more sophisticated view of the change process, and what is required for the profound shifts to happen for people on a course; they defined "Adventure Based Counseling as a group counseling model that uses a carefully sequenced and processed series of experiential activities to elicit behavior change" (p. ix). It is interesting to note that this book advocates for a more "carefully sequenced" group process, while the earlier book states that "a rigid sequence will not serve an Adventure Based Counseling group" (p. 4). These contrasts are reflective of changes in a larger movement towards professionalism.

Adventure Based Counseling/adventure therapy should ultimately be seen as evolving out of Outward Bound as Kurt Hahn's original intent was to bring the adventure and learning of the wilderness experience into the classroom, as well as other indoor facilities. Outward Bound had a major impact on both adventure therapy and wilderness therapy well before these terms were documented and clearly defined.

1974: Association for Experiential Education

The first organization for practitioners of outdoor education, adventure therapy, and wilderness therapy that served individuals involved in Outward Bound, NOLS, Project Adventure and BYU outdoor courses was the Association for Experiential Education (AEE). The organization's first conference took place in Boone, North Caroline in 1974 and was titled "National Conference on Outdoor Pursuits in Higher Education" and was sponsored by Outward Bound International (Miner & Boldt, 1981). AEE started as a loose knit group of experiential educators but has grown into a non-profit professional membership organization of 1555 members located in 13 countries. The Therapeutic Adventure

Professionals Group (TAPG), established at the beginning of AEE, continues to serve an active and involved AEE membership.

It is important to recognize that when this organization began, the definitions of "wilderness therapy" or "Adventure Based Counseling and therapy" had not yet been developed. AEE and TAPG were the first professional organizations for practitioners in the field of wilderness therapy and have been active in researching, educating, and publishing information about the field since the 1970s. It is not until the 1990s that other professional organizations serving the wilderness therapy field emerged. AEE holds regional conferences and one national conference every year. Along with official AEE business, TAPG puts on a pre-conference before each AEE national conference as well as one stand alone, national conference every two years.

In 1994, in recognizing a need and their expertise, AEE developed the first accreditation process for experiential programs for all kinds of standard populations and activities, as well as later for therapeutic populations. In 2013, recognizing their authority and the need for updating best practices, in collaboration with the Outdoor Behavioral Healthcare Council, AEE added more therapeutic detail, support staffing and logistics, additional relevant safety requirements to OBH accreditation designed specifically for Outdoor Behavioral Programs (Association for Experiential Education website, 2014).

1975: Publication of First Document Using the Term "Wilderness Therapy"

The first documented use of the term "wilderness therapy" appears in a 1975 book titled *A Nation Without Prisons: Alternatives to Incarceration,* written by Joseph Nold, then president of Colorado Outward Bound, and Mary Wilpers, a research assistant. The term can be found in their chapter "Wilderness Training as an Alternative to Incarceration." "The essence of 'wilderness therapy' is in this experience: challenge, the overcoming of a seemingly impossible task, the confrontation of fear, a success experience. It is an opportunity to gain self-reliance, to prove one's worth, to define one's manhood. The results are immediate. The task is clear, definable, unavoidable" (p. 155). They describe much of the work done by Outward Bound with "delinquent" youth in the late 1960's and 1970's. They elaborate on how Outward Bound "uses the challenge of wilderness training and service activities to give people a greater sense of their own potentiality, and opportunities for group interaction and leadership, to strengthen their commitment to society…" (p. 155). The majority of the chapter discusses the challenges of a wilderness setting, as well as recidivism research, which all reinforces the use of Outward Bound as a program for "delinquent youth." There is no mention of mental health professionals involved in this first document using the term "wilderness therapy." What this article identifies is that the essence of wilderness therapy is the "challenge" to overcome a seemingly impossible task. The challenge was to teach young people to work together to survive and then be secure in the wilderness without all the accessories or distractions of modern life.

1977: Woodswomen, Inc.

As seen in this section the majority of influences and models in the field were male influenced. In 1977, Woodswomen, Inc., located in Minnesota, was founded by three women – Judith Neimi, Denise Mitten, and Elizabeth Barnard – as a non-profit adventure organization for women and children.

Woodswomen was a unique organization that pioneered several important programmatic aspects of adventure therapy and adventure education from an eco-feminist perspective according to Denise Mitten (personal communication, 9/27/2010). The overarching paradigm at Woodswomen was an ethic of care. From the office to the field, Woodswomen staff reinforced the importance of clients feeling supported and emotionally safe. Consideration of emotional safety is common today, but in the 1970's it was a radical concept. Woodswomen was one of the first organizations to advocate for the emotional safety of participants in all areas of the program.

With this model Woodswomen pioneered working positively with women survivors of abuse. While the majority of adventure therapy programs were using the physical and emotional challenge components found in the Outward Bound model, Woodswomen focused on teaching participants stress management while on trips. This is common practice today but not in the early days of the field. The organization closed in 1999 but the philosophy and theories behind it were elaborated on in the book *Wilderness Therapy for Women: The Power of Adventure* (1994), edited by Cole, Erdman & Rothblum.

1978: Publication of Larry Wells' *A Guide to Wilderness Therapy Programs*

Another early document that used the term "wilderness therapy" was printed in 1978 and written by Larry Wells in a self-published pamphlet titled *A Guide to Wilderness Therapy Programs*. In the document, he explained, "I receive many inquiries as to how to conduct outdoor rehabilitation programs for delinquents, how to start a program, where to find funding, etc. As a result I've published this booklet not only to give some pointers on starting a program and conducting one, but also information on working with troubled youth" (p. 4). In the section on requisite staff skills, he described, "staff must be first aid qualified" and "be trained or certified in wilderness skills and if at all possible, have counseling experience and training" (p. 38). He encouraged programs to have a design that provides for growth in three areas for the participants: "mental, physical and spiritual" (p. 9). He also encouraged three phases in a wilderness therapy program: "Impact – a time when the student is stripped of all material facades or relating tools to which they are accustomed… Student Expeditions – a time when, as a team, the students accomplish a teamwork challenge… Solo – a time to be alone to internalize…" (p. 11). The phases in this document are a directly reflection of the BYU 480 model.

In his pamphlet, Wells espouses the use of "outdoor rehabilitation programs as the most successful approach for delinquent behavior youth" (p. 5). There are no references to having mental health professionals in assisting with the process yet he did encourage the use of "transactional analysis" and the need to help the family in working with delinquent youth (p. 16). At the end of the pamphlet, Wells provided a compilation of forms for starting one's own wilderness therapy program, as well as areas in the Western United States to operate. This unique document is one of the earliest to describe a primitive skills model and one of the first to include, in its title, "Wilderness Therapy." Some of what is written in this document is still being practiced today.

Larry Wells has only been identified in two documents (Russell & Hendee, 2000, White, 2011) as critical to the evolution of the field of wilderness therapy yet his profound influence can be identified in several ways, including for starting one of the earliest not-for-profit primitive skills wilderness therapy programs, Expedition Outreach; for helping launch the first for-profit program for adjudicated youth, VisionQuest; for opening one of the first wilderness therapy organizations specifically for substance abusing youth, Wilderness Conquest (later referred to as Wilderness Quest); and for publishing the first guide intending to support the expansion of wilderness therapy programs. Wells would also assist the start-up of numerous other primitive skills based wilderness therapy organizations in the West.

Wells' "how-to" pamphlet for starting a wilderness therapy program was sold by the Association of Experiential Education at its national and regional conferences. One of the many people to buy one of Wells' pamphlets was the director of the Santa Fe Mountain Center, Richard "Rocky" Kimball.

1979: Santa Fe Mountain Center

The Santa Fe Mountain Center evolved out of the state of New Mexico's Bureau of Mental Health and the Health and Environment Department to become a private nonprofit organization in 1979. This transition was facilitated by Richard Kimball, Ph.D. Kimball had been an instructor at Colorado Outward Bound in the early 1970s and was later awarded a fellowship to attend University of Colorado where he received his Ph.D. in education. His first job, after receiving his doctorate, was for the state of New Mexico. Kimball explains the state's initial objective: "What we were trying to do was to inject Outward Bound into the schools and the mental health centers" (R. Kimball, personal communication, August 18, 2010). Kimball recognized that the state's program might be eliminated based on annual budget concerns. He believed that the only way for the program to survive was to become independent from the state and that it would have to innovate through private initiatives. This created a unique organizational model of a non-profit emerging out of a state agency.

Instead of hiring former Outward Bound instructors like himself, Kimball focused on hiring professionals with mental health backgrounds who possessed strong outdoor and group skills. The Santa Fe Mountain Center staff encouraged the organization to broaden its focus, beyond youth at risk, to work with other vulnerable populations. This broadened clientele allowed Santa Fe Mountain Center to grow even during economic challenges. What was unique about Santa Fe Mountain Center was this ability to adapt to the needs of a variety of mental health populations and difficult economic times. In a time when many nonprofits in the wilderness therapy field have closed, the Santa Fe Mountain Center still thrives. Two years after the founding of Santa Fe Mountain Center, the School of Urban and Wilderness Survival was founded.

1981: School of Urban and Wilderness Survival (SUWS)

The first for-profit, private-pay primitive skills-based wilderness therapy program (initially known as a Wilderness Experience Program) opened in Idaho as the School of Urban and Wilderness Survival, or SUWS (pronounced "SOOS"), in 1981 by L. Jay Mitchell and George Church. Mitchell, another former BYU 480 student, approached Larry Olsen, who had departed from BYU, to develop the philosophy, curriculum, and staff training for SUWS. SUWS also employed Larry Wells to assist in the primitive skills programming while he also conducted trips in Northwest Washington and Central Idaho. In the beginning, the organization did not employ psychotherapists. The 21-day program was based on the BYU Survival Class, but was focused on teenagers who had been in trouble at home or school. In the first years of the program, participants would go out on 21-day treks while learning primitive skills in order to cook food and build shelters. Within six years, SUWS became a thriving program due in part to the active national marketing campaign by its directors.

SUWS is a critical organization for several reasons, including: the program was the first to take escorted adolescents (unwilling participants brought to the program against their will but with parent's permission), it had a national focus enrolling adolescents from all over the country, and it became notably profitable (L. Woodbury, personal communication, July 7, 2010). Unlike earlier organizations, which had contracted with state or local social services or corrections, SUWS focused on private-pay participants – and their financial success enticed many to enter the private-pay field. The SUWS program was purchased from Mitchell and Church in June of 1994 for an undisclosed sum by College Health Enterprises (later renamed Aspen Education Group).

During the summer of 2000, Aspen Education Group established "SUWS of the Carolinas" in North Carolina and so its predecessor henceforth would be referred to as "SUWS of Idaho." During the summer of 2013, the Aspen Education Group/CRC group would close several wilderness therapy programs including SUWS of Idaho as, according to president of CRC Health, Susan Cambria, at the time, "[it] had become abundantly clear that the current market... [did] not support... maintaining our [CRC's] entire network of therapeutic programs." ("Aspen Education Group Closes Five Programs,"2010).

Although SUWS of Idaho closed, SUWS of the Carolinas is still operating. Several organizations inspired by SUWS or started with former SUWS staff will be revealed later in this chapter. Another long-standing private-pay program opened shortly after SUWS; and its model included licensed substance abuse counselors but its influence was not tied to BYU 480.

1983: Wilderness Treatment Center

The Wilderness Treatment Center is one of the first and longest running wilderness therapy programs in the United States. It is also the first to have licensed chemical dependency counselors working with participants while out on wilderness expeditions. The program opened in 1983 as an inpatient substance abuse program with John Brekke, a certified chemical dependency counselor, as the director. Before opening Wilderness Treatment Center, Brekke had combined the Minnesota Model of Chemical Dependency Treatment (developed by Hazelden Alcohol and Drug Treatment Center) with Outward Bound type expeditions. Brekke took adjudicated, substance-abusing youth from the Swan River Youth Forest Camp out on wilderness trips. Brekke was influenced by Outward Bound (he had participated in several Outward Bound courses), as well as his friend, Paul Petzoldt, the mountaineer and founder of National Outdoor Leadership School and Wilderness Education Association. Brekke had journeyed with Petzoldt, and other outdoor experiential leaders, to a two-week climb of the Grand Teton to develop the treatment curriculum for Wilderness Treatment Center (Brekke, 2005).

Wilderness Treatment Center is a private-pay program for adolescent males and has always been licensed as a sixty-day inpatient substance abuse center, with the first thirty days of intensive substance abuse counseling followed by a twenty-eight-day wilderness expedition, returning back to a rustic base just outside Glacier National Park for debriefing of the experience. Sadly, Brekke would die unexpectedly in the fall of 2013 but Wilderness Treatment Center still stands as the longest program of its style in the country. Its model of including substance abuse counselors in the field with participants would later be replicated in Oregon.

This program and its history are briefly outlined in a 2005 online article, "Therapist in the Woods," by John Brekke, the founder of Wilderness Treatment Center.

1988: Catherine Freer Wilderness Expeditions

Four years after the opening of Wilderness Treatment Center, a multitude of private-pay programs opened in the West. The majority, unlike Wilderness Treatment Center, did not include mental health professionals on staff and all were initially not licensed (Utah did not have licensure until July of 1990). Another exception to this wild west expansion of outdoor treatment was offered by the Catherine Freer Wilderness Survival School (later renamed Catherine Freer Wilderness Therapy Expeditions), a 1988 Oregon program licensed as a residential alcohol and drug treatment program; Catherine Freer Wilderness Therapy Expeditions employed licensed substance abuse counselors on all trips (Woodbury, 1991a). This organization was co-founded by Rob Cooley, Ph.D., and its mountaineering style was influenced by the organization's namesake, Catherine Freer, who was an established mountaineer and friend of Cooley's. Freer was initially involved in the start-up of the organization but died in a tragic climbing accident, according to the program's website. Catherine Freer's Wilderness Therapy Expeditions was similar to Wilderness Treatment Center, as it had licensed counselors in the field but unlike Wilderness Treatment Center in that the students were never in a residence, since the program took place completely in the wilderness. Catherine Freer Wilderness Therapy Expeditions closed in 2012, "due to changes in insurance regulations and policies, [meaning] few insurance companies… pay for the program." Cooley continued, "That, combined with the lingering recession, limited the number of families that the program could serve and contributed to the decision to close the program" (Cooley retires…Catherine Freer Closes, 2012).

Wilderness Treatment Center and the Catherine Freer Wilderness Therapy Expeditions aside, the following private for-profit organizations that opened in 1988 can be directly traced to BYU 480.

1988: Anasazi Foundation

In 1987, Larry Olsen departed the SUWS organization and, within a year, started the Anasazi Foundation by joining again with Ezekiel Sanchez in Arizona. Initially, Anasazi was a for-profit organization. However, after the first year, Olsen and Sanchez decided that they wanted the organization to be available to all, independent of the ability to pay, so they reorganized and became a not-for-profit. What was significant about the Anasazi Foundation is that it became a non-profit primitive skills based wilderness therapy organization when so many for-profits were opening, and it actively sought licensure in order to get insurance reimbursement for services to lower the costs for families (White, 2008). Anasazi and Wilderness Treatment Center are two of the few programs of this era that are still in existence today. (Anasazi's story will be told by its co-founder Ezekial Sanchez, in the second section of this book.)

1988: Wilderness Quest

In 1988, Larry Wells opened Wilderness Conquest (later renamed Wilderness Quest) as a for-profit primitive skills-based wilderness therapy program specifically for substance abusing teens in Monticello, Utah. What is significant about Wilderness Quest is that it was the first for-profit primitive skills based organization specifically for substance-abusing participants. Wells described the program's focus:

> "After doing Expedition Outreach, on and off for years, I went on to start my first private pay program, Wilderness Conquest (later renamed Wilderness Quest). Our program was focused on Twelve Steps. We just fit with that because that's what we as a family were. Our whole thing, before we had any of this other stuff, was spiritual and my belief was that you've got to replace the drugs with something. A

spiritual connection is part of the Twelve Steps {of Alcoholics Anonymous}. I mean you've got to replace it with something you can trust and connect with, and you've got to deal with the students/clients with respect, love and concern.

At Wilderness Quest, we used expeditions and wilderness activities that, upon accomplishing, increase student's self-esteem, their self-confidence, which in turn, because they're having success and responsibility, increases their maturity. You have to pre-load wilderness activities and, at the same time, you have to pre-load them in group discussions. We set the tone and what the expectations are and then you have to debrief the experience or post-process so you help them understand what they have accomplished. That part of it is talking, the pre- and the post, but the activity that actually changes thought and behavior is the wilderness experiences of some kind. Whether it is just cranking a fire out with a fire bow and being all excited that you've achieved that, you know, and learning how to do that." (White, 2011, pg. 162-163)

Wells would sell his interest in Wilderness Quest in 2005 and the program would close its doors in 2012.

1988: Wilderness Academy (aka: Aspen Achievement Academy)

Wilderness Academy, later renamed Aspen Achievement Academy, was co-founded in 1988 by Dr. Keith Hooker, Doug Cloward, Madolyn Liebing, Ph.D., and Doug Nelson (faculty at BYU and the founder of Boulder Outdoor Survival School), all former BYU 480 students or instructors (Stednitz, 1991). What is significant about Aspen Achievement Academy is that it was the first primitive skills-based wilderness therapy organization to employ in its services a full-time doctoral level, licensed psychologist, Dr. Liebing, and a physician, Dr. Hooker. Liebing provided individual therapy and psychological evaluations to participants in the field. Liebing was the first licensed psychologist to work in a primitive skills wilderness therapy organization and would later start The Journey (see second section). Hooker provided medical oversight of participants.

Wilderness Academy would become the first state-licensed wilderness therapy program in Utah.

The addition of a licensed mental health professional, as well as a clinical focus, created an upsurge in referrals to Aspen. The organization would be sold by its original founders and change its name to Aspen Achievement Academy; it would later be featured in a book about the field called *Shouting at the Sky: Troubled Teens and the Promise of the Wild* by Gary Ferguson (1999) and in the third season of the British Reality Television series titled *Brat Camp*. Several other clinically-focused, primitive skills based wilderness therapy organizations, including RedCliff Ascent, Open Sky Wilderness Therapy, Second Nature and Legacy Outdoor Adventures (all featured in the next section), would be founded, or helped with the startup process, by former Aspen staff, in the 1990s and 2000s. Aspen Achievement Academy would "discontinue operations" in 2011 due to "the reduced demand for therapeutic schools and programs in today's economy" according to a 2011 press release by Phil Hershman, President of Aspen Education Group (Aspen Education Group to Restructure Programs, 2011).

By the late 1980s and 1990s, private, for-profit, primitive skills-based wilderness therapy programs for adolescents exploded in the West, as well as other parts of the country. This rapid expansion of the field was due, in part, to increased demands for adolescent treatment from desperate parents. This desperation came with the closure of many adolescent inpatient psychiatric hospitals and substance abuse treatment centers due to the adoption of managed health care by insurance companies (Santa, 2007). With this expansion came controversy brought on by those who were enticed to the field by the potential high profits and low startup costs. This is best personified by the Challenger Foundation.

1988: The Challenger Foundation

One of the most extreme and documented cases of abuse and neglect in a wilderness therapy organization occurred at the Challenger Foundation, founded by Steve Cartisano. One of the first articles about this organization, as well as other abusive organizations, was titled "Loving Them to Death," published in *Outside Magazine* (October 1995) and written by the then little-known mountaineer and journalist, Jon Krakauer. The opening sentences of Krakauer's article sets the tone: "It's the 'wilderness experience' at its most extreme – rehabilitation of wayward teenagers delivered with the in-your-face discipline of a boot camp. But in the past five years at least four young people have died, the victims of alleged beatings, starvation, and emotional abuse, and the so-called therapy is looking more like murder" (Krakauer, 1995, p. 72). Krakauer focused primarily on primitive skills-based wilderness therapy programs in the West and particularly those related to BYU. The document points to the culture of abuse in the Challenger Foundation and how this culture would be subsequently adopted by other individuals, who had worked at the Challenger Foundation, who would start wilderness therapy organizations where other deaths would occur.

In the beginning of the article, Krakauer (1995) laid out the origins of the field, including Outward Bound, and was the first to document how the field was influenced by BYU and Larry Dean Olsen, as well as how wilderness therapy programs grew in the West. He stated that the main differences between Outward Bound and BYU 480 was that BYU is closely affiliated with the Church of Jesus Christ of Latter-day Saints (LDS) and that many graduates of BYU courses established similar programs across the West (p. 76). The majority of the *Outside Magazine* article focuses on Cartisano, a former BYU student and military man, as the person who made wilderness therapy a high-profit business and promoted an approach of dealing with students by an "in-your-face" style of confrontation.

Krakauer (1995) revealed that Cartisano, who as an Air Force service member was an instructor in the elite paratrooper survival school, converted to the LDS faith while in the service, and, after leaving the service, attended BYU (p. 77). Cartisano did not receive a degree while at BYU but worked briefly as an instructor "in one of the school's wilderness courses" (no documents verify he attended BYU 480) and "thereby found his calling" (p. 77). Cartisano started the Challenger Foundation in 1987 in Hawaii. In January of 1988, he brought the program to Utah where he began to charge $15,900 for a two-month wilderness therapy program while other programs were charging $500 for a one-month course (p. 77). Cartisano had assistance in starting the Challenger Foundation by employing both Larry Wells and Doug Nelson in the startup phase, yet both would quickly separate themselves from the Challenger Foundation and Cartisano (Roche, 1989).

Cartisano, a brilliant promoter, hired a publicist and went on a national marketing campaign, including many television talk shows that highlighted the impact of the Challenger Foundation. According to Krakauer (1995), "like Outward Bound, most Mormon-run wilderness schools offered kids tough challenges but generally treated them with care and sensitivity. Cartisano disdained this approach as too touchy-feely. Instead, he ran the Challenger Foundation with the in-your-face discipline of a boot camp" (p. 77). In 1990, a death occurred at the Challenger Foundation; a 16-year-old girl, named Kristen Chase, collapsed while hiking in 100°F weather after staff ignored her complaints, thinking she was "faking" it (p. 80). Kristen Chase died of dehydration. Cartisano and other program staff were charged with negligent homicide and abuse but were later acquitted by a jury (p. 80). The Challenger Foundation was closed down by the State of Utah in 1990.

What is significant about the Challenger Foundation is that it is the most documented example of an abusive culture in a wilderness therapy program and that this culture of treating participants as objects would be replicated in other programs where abuse and deaths would also occur (Gregory, 2000; Krakauer, 1995; Morganstern, 1995; Szalavitz, 2006). Because of Cartisano and the staff of the Challenger Foundation's actions, the State of Utah recognized the need to regulate wilderness therapy programs in 1990. This was the second death in a Utah-based wilderness therapy organization and, even after state licensure, this did not stop other abusive organizations from springing up. Many of the deaths that occurred in wilderness therapy programs at that time were connected to the Challenger Foundation, as several former Challenger Foundation staff went on to start other organizations, such as Summit Quest and North Star Expeditions, where avoidable deaths would occur.

1990: Summit Quest

Before the death at the Challenger Foundation, the former admissions director of the Challenger Foundation, Gayle Palmer, left the program to start her own program, named Summit Quest. Palmer had no outdoor experience or training in psychology but had seen the profits of the Challenger Foundation and decided to open her own program

(Szalavitz, 2006, p. 101). On the first expedition of Summit Quest, in May of 1990, a 15-year-old girl, Michelle Sutton, would die from dehydration while staff ignored her (Szalavitz, 2006, p. 102). After the death, Cartisano reportedly said that a tragedy like that "could never happen at Challenger"; two months later, Kristen Chase died at the Challenger Foundation (Szalavitz, 2006, p. 102). Another death of a participant occurred at North Star Expeditions in 1994 and this death, and author Krakaur's provocative exposé, would later bring about calls for federal regulation of wilderness therapy organizations as well as the galvanization of wilderness therapy organizations to create best practice standards for safety, and treatment.

1990: North Star Expeditions

A 1992 press release by North Star Expeditions described their organization as a 63-day wilderness-based program licensed by the State of Utah since 1990. The organization's philosophy statement was "Stripping away current societal influences and going back to the rigors faced by our homesteading families and pioneers, a scant 100 years ago, young people begin to see the world and their place in it differently than before. Re-discovering the values and foundation of character instilled by their parents" (Woodbury, 1992). What is significant about this organization is it was founded by people who had previously worked at the Challenger Foundation, Lance Jagger and Bill Henry, who continued the same culture of confrontation of and "breaking down" the participants. The difference was that North Star Expeditions was now licensed by the State of Utah, and that it had a licensed mental health counselor (a clinical social worker) on staff. Yet, "therapy at North Star consisted almost exclusively of intimidation, deprivation, and military-style discipline," (Krakauer, 1995, p. 80).

In March of 1994, a 16-year-old boy named Aaron Bacon was brought from his home in Arizona, by North Star Expeditions staff, to Utah. During his first weeks in the program, Bacon, repeatedly complained of feeling ill, was unable to keep down food or water, and lost a considerable about of weight. Bacon was neglected by the staff who accused him of "faking it" and subsequently died in large part because of the program culture of in-your-face discipline (Krakauer, 1995). Bacon's death was from complications of a perforated ulcer and subsequent infection. In a photo taken shortly before he died, he looks emaciated and quite ill but he was not helped by the staff of North Star until it was too late. North Star was subsequently closed by the state but the legacy of Bacon's death continues, as Bob and Sally Bacon, parents of Aaron Bacon, have been tireless advocates for federal regulations (in addition to states' oversight) of wilderness therapy programs since the death of their son. In 2009, a film would be released about their son's death titled *Aaron Bacon*.

The tragic legacy of the Challenger Foundation and North Star Expeditions reappeared in Oregon when the individual who conducted the "parental guidance seminar" for the North Star organization, Greg Bodenhamer (Woodbury, 1992), would subsequently start a wilderness therapy program in 1998 called Obsidian Trails. Obsidian Trails and Bodenhamer would also employ former staff from North Star Expeditions (the son and wife of the founder, Bill Henry) (Gregory, 2000). In 2000, a student would die at Obsidian Trails while being restrained and the program would later close (Schutt, 2000). The deaths and abuses in wilderness therapy organizations during the 1980s and the 1990s served as a catalyst for greater research and increased publications about the field. This has been evidenced by the flurry of books and articles that were published in the 1990s and the start of several professional organizations.

1993: Publication of *Adventure Therapy: Theory, Research, and Practice*

In 1993, Michael Gass, Ph.D., a professor of kinesiology at the University of New Hampshire, edited a book entitled *Adventure Therapy: Therapeutic Applications of Adventure Programming*. In this book, Gass parses the field of adventure therapy into three "types" and, in Chapter 1 titled "Foundations of Adventure Therapy," he identifies the primary influences of each type of programming. "It is interesting to note that the use of adventure therapy has evolved into three general areas of implementation" (Gass, 1993, p. 9). The three areas outlined are: wilderness therapy, adventure-based therapy, and long-term residential camping. In this paragraph, he includes these three types of models, elaborates with program examples, and puts the models under the umbrella of the term adventure therapy:

> **Wilderness therapy** – here, the therapeutic experience occurs in remote wilderness setting and tends to consist of small-group (8-15), multiple-day (e.g., 24 days), round-the-clock intervention. Outward Bound programs and adapted Outward Bound programs (e.g., Santa Fe Mountain Center) were the primary innovators of this type of therapeutic programming.
>
> **Adventure-based therapy** – here, the therapeutic experience occurs at or very close to the therapeutic facility of the client. These programs tend to be in-patient programs where patients are in multiple-day treatment programs, and adventure therapy is only one part of the therapeutic intervention being used…. While such programs possess the same origin as wilderness therapy programs with Outward Bound, their expansion can be linked to a number of programs like Project Adventure.
>
> **Long-term residential camping** – based on the values inherent in wilderness camping (e.g. Loughmiller, 1965), this form of outdoor programming focuses on placing adolescents or other adjudicated populations into outdoor camps (e.g., Eckerd Foundation Camps, Dallas Salesmanship Club Camp) or on mobile travel units (e.g., wagon trains, sail training on clipper ships). (Gass, 1993, p. 9-10)

This chapter is significant as it identifies the critical influences in definitions and models in the evolvement of the field.

Richard Kimball (previously mentioned re: the Santa Fe Mountain Center) and Stephen Bacon (1993), two Ph.D.'s who had been worked at Outward Bound, would publish a chapter in *Adventure Therapy: Therapeutic Applications of Adventure Programming* that described "Wilderness Therapy" as "difficult to define the process [of] precisely" yet there are "activities and processes that characterize the approach" (p. 117-118). Their chapter acknowledges the Kurt Hahn DNA throughout wilderness therapy but they elaborate further that activities and processes that characterize wilderness therapy include a group process because "there is no such thing as 'individual' wilderness therapy" (p. 118). They explain that wilderness therapy includes a series of challenges that incrementally increase to a higher level of difficulty which may, to the participant, seem insurmountable; the main idea in the challenges is that they are "perceived as high risk but are low in actual risk" (p. 118). They state that the wilderness therapy process should be in the wilderness or in "unfamiliar environments" and should "employ therapy techniques, time alone for reflection and journal writing, psychoeducational-techniques, individual counseling, staff modeling, and self-disclosure" (p. 118). Interestingly, this definition does not include having mental health professionals as part of the wilderness therapy staff. When this definition of wilderness therapy was printed, as seen in this section, it reflected the state of the majority of the field which was staffed generally by outdoor educators who had little or no clinical training; there was no credentialing associated with the field, and there was little to no family involvement. Shortly thereafter, Powch (1994) would question the definition of "wilderness therapy."

1994: Publication of "Wilderness Therapy: What Makes it Empowering for Women?"

In 1994, Irene Powch, a doctoral student, published a chapter in the journal *Women and Therapy* entitled "Wilderness Therapy: What Makes it Empowering for Women?" In the chapter, she references that "historical roots of the common conception of Wilderness Therapy lie in the original Outward Bound model" (p. 13). Powch does not mention BYU 480 or primitive skills organizations. She states that other terms such as "adventure-based therapy" and "ropes courses" are inaccurately used "synonymously for the term 'wilderness therapy'." To remedy this issue, she insists that wilderness therapy "must occur in a wilderness setting and that the wilderness must be approached with a therapeutic goal in mind" (p. 14). She explains, "I do not dispute that therapy can occur in settings other than the wilderness, but I would not call it wilderness therapy." She reinforces the view of wilderness therapy taking place in remote outside settings. The Powch article is important not only for its refinement of the definition of wilderness therapy and inclusion of the therapeutic goals but also for exploring wilderness therapy for women for its effectiveness in dealing with trauma and the spiritual aspects of wilderness therapy. Powch's article would be reprinted in a book titled *Wilderness Therapy for Women: The Power of Adventure* (1994), edited by Ellen Cole, Eve Erdman, and Esther Rothblum. This is an excellent book about wilderness therapy for women by women but is focused primarily on adults. At the same time, another book with "Wilderness Therapy" in the title was published that focused primarily on wilderness therapy for youth.

1994: Publication of *Wilderness Therapy: Foundation, Theories, and Research*

In 1994, Jennifer Davis-Berman and Dene Berman, two Ph.D.'s who have written and researched extensively on wilderness therapy, authored *Wilderness Therapy: Foundations, Theories, and Research* (1994). They define wilderness therapy as "the use of traditional therapy techniques, especially in group therapy, in an out-of-doors setting, utilizing outdoor adventure pursuits and other activities to enhance personal growth" (p. 13). They explain that wilderness therapy "involves the careful selection of potential candidates based on a clinical assessment and the creation of an individual treatment plan for each participant" (p. 13). They further state that group psychotherapy should be included by "qualified professionals" (p. 140) without further definition. Davis-Berman and Berman's first book helped to define wilderness therapy and provided both theoretical understanding and the first documented history of the field as well as reviewed some of its early research.

In 2008, Jennifer Davis-Berman and Dene Berman authored *The Promise of Wilderness Therapy* (2008) which would be published as "[a] comprehensive guide to how and why wilderness therapy can be a solution for at-risk youth who aren't making headway in traditional therapy" (Davis-Berman and Berman, 2008, book cover). This book is written for parents who are looking for wilderness therapy programs in which to enroll their adolescent. Davis-Berman and Berman (2008) are explicit in their statements that "group and individual therapy is the heart of the wilderness therapy program" and "therapy should be provided by qualified fully licensed mental health professionals" (p. 15). Davis-

Berman and Berman's advice to parents is reflective of the current state of the field.

Another book, published in 1999, turned the focus from academic justifications and data regarding wilderness therapy and instead, captured the essence of primitive skills wilderness expeditions in a more lyrical prose, highlighting the relationships between staff (primarily focusing on Instructors) and students who did therapeutic work in wilderness settings.

1999: Publication of *Shouting at the Sky*

The first book written about wilderness therapy, by someone not involved with the field, was *Shouting at the Sky* by Gary Ferguson (1999). Ferguson, who had written dozens of books on nature and science, became interested in the field after coming upon an article about success rates in wilderness therapy. He approached Aspen Achievement Academy and asked to work as a field staff member while writing about his and others' experiences. In his book, Ferguson describes Aspen's approach to working with adolescents in the wilderness; the variety of issues that brought adolescents to be enrolled in the program, and the challenges of being a staff working in wilderness therapy.

This book is an excellent resource for those who know little about the wilderness therapy field and want to get a sense of what happens around the campfire, in field sessions and during conflicts and how the group grows and protects their sense of community. Ferguson did not paint a completely positive view of the wilderness therapy field; he wrote that "... [w]ilderness therapy in general has been equated with... [Bacon's] tragic, senseless death ever since" and that an educational consultant advised him that "good programs are the exception and not the rule" (p. 15). The tragic, often indefensible deaths of participants would spur practitioners to create best-practice organizations to cull the abusive and rogue programs from the growing association of professional organizations.

1994: Professional Organization: National Association of Therapeutic Wilderness Camps

The National Association of Therapeutic Wilderness Camps (NATWC), later referred to as the National Association of Therapeutic Wilderness

Camping, came together in 1994 at Black Mountain, North Carolina (R. McClintock, personal communication, March 8, 2010). The first conference attendees included a diverse group of organizations and people from different parts of the country. Those attending included Larry Olsen and Ezekiel Sanchez, from Anasazi, as well as other representatives from the Dallas Salesmanship Club and Three Springs. According to Rick McClintock, former director of NATWC, "The NATWC group was focused on the impact that the Aaron Bacon incident in the West had on Outdoor programming, and was looking to set some standards of operations" (R. McClintock, personal communication, March 8, 2010). The group met with the Council on Accreditation (CoA) to help create standards for licensure/accreditation of programs in the field. NATWC, at one time, represented over 50 therapeutic wilderness programs and had yearly conferences. NATWC would quietly disband as a professional organization in late 2012. In its place, the rise of the Outdoor Behavioral Healthcare Council cannot be overstated.

1997: Professional Organization: Outdoor Behavioral Healthcare Council

The Outdoor Behavioral Healthcare Council (OBH Council) was founded in 1997 when representatives from a handful of wilderness treatment programs (Anasazi, Aspen Achievement Academy, RedCliff Ascent, SUWS of Idaho, and Catherine Freer Wilderness) joined to collaborate and to share best practices (OBHC website). What is interesting to note is that four of the founding member organizations are primitive skills-based organizations and of the five founding organizations, only RedCliff Ascent and Anasazi are still in operation. The council founded the Outdoor Behavioral Healthcare Research Cooperative (OBHRC) and has funded numerous research studies on the effectiveness of wilderness therapy. The rationale for the use of the term "Outdoor Behavioral Healthcare" versus "Wilderness Therapy," and the clearer definition of OBH, is offered by Keith Russell and John Hendee (2000). The OBH Council also now sponsors and organizes the Wilderness Therapy Symposium, which includes the latest research and best practices within the field. A more in depth chapter on the history of OBH Council is in the second section of this book.

1999: Professional Organization: National Association of Therapeutic Schools and Programs (NATSAP)

Responding to the uproar caused by deaths in programs that seemed more boot camp than therapeutic, another group of program folks established the National Association of Therapeutic Schools and Programs (NATSAP) in 1999 as a trade organization, "to serve as an advocate and resource for innovative schools and programs, which devote themselves to society's need for the effective care and education of struggling young people" (Santa, 2007). NATSAP has over 142 member programs some of which are wilderness therapy organizations, the majority of which are for-profit treatment programs. The organization currently requires that all members be either licensed by their state and/or by a national accrediting organization, such as the Council on Accreditation (COA) or the Joint Commission of Accreditation of Healthcare Organizations (JCOA). The organization has a yearly national conference, numerous regional conferences, and puts out a journal of research related to the field.

In 2004, as more organizations, academics, and writers focused on the field of wilderness therapy, it became inevitable that the field would emerge into popular culture via television. Before that, researchers started to question what the field was about and focused on an accurate definition of the field.

2000: Technical Report: "Outdoor Behavioral Healthcare"

Keith Russell and John Hendee (2000), two Ph.D. researchers and professors at the University of Idaho, encouraged a shift away from the term "Wilderness Therapy" to a more descriptive term referred to as "Outdoor Behavioral Healthcare." They defined Outdoor Behavioral Healthcare (OBH) as "…an emerging intervention and treatment in mental health practice to help adolescents overcome emotional, adjustment, addictions, and psychological problems. OBH programs utilize elements of wilderness therapy to help adolescents and their families, which include: immersion in an unfamiliar environment, group living with peers, individual and group therapy sessions, and educational curricula including backcountry travel and wilderness living skills, all designed to reveal and address problem behaviors and foster personal and social responsibility and emotional growth of adolescent clients." (Russell & Hendee, 2000, p. 3)

Outdoor Behavioral Healthcare is "specifically aimed at changing destructive, dysfunctional or problem behavior in clients through clinically supervised therapy, therapeutic activities, and an educational program in outdoor settings" (Russell & Hendee, 2000, p. 8). What is significant of Russell and Hendee's (2000) updated definition is its development after tracing the field's historical roots; they were the first, in scholarly literature, to identify the critical influence of primitive skills programs on the field of wilderness therapy.

Russell and Hendee (2000) cited seven historical influences on the evolution of the field were:

1. Therapeutic camping (Dallas Salesmanship Club)

2. Wilderness challenge model (Outward Bound)

3. Primitive skills programs (BYU 480)

4. Adjudicated programs (VisionQuest)

5. Professional organizations (AEE, OBHIC)

6. Scholarly influences (Davis-Berman and Berman, Russell and Hendee)

7. Insurance and licensure recognition (Anasazi) (p.35)

Although their historical review is limited to ten pages, it was the most inclusive document about the many influences on the field, including BYU 480 as well as Olsen, Sanchez, and Wells. The document does not include earlier influences such as Camp Chocorua, Boy Scouting, or the first therapeutic summer camps. In 2003, the first of what was to become an annual event identified and paid homage to the early founders of the primitive skills movement.

2003: Clan of the Hand

RedCliff Ascent, a primitive-skills based wilderness therapy organization founded in 1993 located in Enterprise, Utah, would start a tradition of honoring those who helped shape the primitive-skills based wilderness therapy field. Scott Schill, now RedCliff Ascent's Executive Director (and former Wilderness Academy staff), proposed an event to honor some of the 'old timers' in wilderness therapy. As part of this ceremony, inductees were asked to put their handprints on the wall of a kiva (a Native American underground room used for spiritual ceremonies) that was built in their honor. This was the first wilderness therapy "Hall of Fame."

The first five to be honored in 2003 were Larry Dean Olsen and Ezekiel Sanchez, Doug Nelson, Larry Wells and David Wescott (S. Schill, personal communication, September 25, 2010). Since '03, six more inducted have placed their hands on the wall and joined the Clan: Dr. Keith Hooker, Kay Harris, Ken Stettler, George Church, David Holladay, and Karen Wells (married to Larry Wells). This writer came upon this undocumented ceremony when completing the interviews for his doctoral dissertation titled, "Stories from the Elders: Chronicles and Narratives from the Early Years of Wilderness Therapy" (White, 2011).

RedCliff Ascent's first Clan of the Hand ceremony focused on honoring the past. A year later, RedCliff Ascent would participate in introducing the primitive skills model to an international television audience (RedCliff Ascent is also one of the programs highlighted in the second section of this book).

2004: Reality Television: *Brat Camp*

Wilderness therapy was first introduced to popular culture in a reality television series entitled *Brat Camp,* which aired on US, British, and Australian airwaves in 2004 (Jones, 2006, p. 30). The first series followed a group of British teenage adolescents' lives before, during, and after enrollment at RedCliff Ascent. This was the second time that RedCliff Ascent had been featured on television with their first exposure being in a 2001 (A&E Investigative Report titled *Teen Wilderness Camps: Therapy or Punishment?*). The commercials for

Brat Camp stated "problem British teenagers brought to a desert wilderness therapy program to address their problems through primitive living and therapy." There are a variety of ethical questions related to filming adolescents in treatment, as well as the use of the term "Brat Camp," that were explored in an article by Jennifer Jones (2006) titled "When the Cameras are Rolling – a Utah Wilderness Therapy Program Faced Conflicts When it Became a Reality TV Series Subject." RedCliff Ascent officials were generally happy with *Brat Camp* but did not like the name and thought the program focused too much on the primitive survival skills and not enough on the therapy (Jones, 2006, p. 34). Because of *Brat Camp*'s success RedCliff Ascent was offered to do another segment but declined. Two other wilderness therapy programs, Aspen Achievement Academy and SageWalk, agreed to be filmed in the subsequent segments of the series, however both programs are no longer in operation.

2007: Congressional Investigation

With notoriety from recent suspicious deaths and now with increasing public awareness due to these television shows, Representative George Miller (D-CA) in 2007 began investigations and called upon the Government Accountability Office (GAO) to investigate the private-pay therapeutic industry, and specifically several wilderness therapy programs, as well as other residential programs.

The abuse and deaths of program participants first reported in Krakauer's (1995) national magazine article and other regional newspaper articles (Gregory 2000; Morganstern, 1995) would be later followed by a book written by Maia Szalavitz (2006), a journalist, in *Help at Any Cost*. Szalavitz' book not only harshly reviews and questions the effectiveness of wilderness therapy in general but also casts doubts on the effectiveness of for-profit adolescent residential treatment programs in general. Szalavitz (2006) studied the deaths at the Challenger Foundation, Summit Quest, and the State of Utah-licensed North Star Expeditions, and she encouraged federal regulations of programs: "As I write [2006], there is still no federal regulation to protect children in privately run wilderness programs and boot camps" (p. 120). The culmination of these articles, books, and the advocacy of former participants and parents whose children died while enrolled in wilderness therapy programs, was a 2007 US Government

Accountability Office investigation of the field of wilderness therapy, as well as other residential treatment programs for youth.

In 2007, a document was released by the GAO titled *Residential Treatment Programs – Concerns Regarding Abuse and Death in Certain Programs for Troubled Youth* (Government Accounting Office, 2007). The report starts with, "GAO found thousands of allegations of abuse, some of which involved death, at residential treatment programs across the country and in American-owned and American operated facilities abroad between the years 1990 and 2007" (p. 1). In the report the "GAO also examined, in greater detail, 10 closed or criminal cases from 1990 through 2004 where a teenager died while enrolled in a private program. GAO found significant evidence of ineffective management in most of the 10 cases, with program leaders neglecting the needs of program participants and staff" (p. 1). Although the investigation was not only about wilderness therapy programs, it should be noted that eight of the ten cases of death, reviewed by the GAO, were in wilderness therapy organizations. In May of 2008, the GAO published a follow-up document titled *Residential Facilities: Improved Data and Enhanced Oversight Would Help Safeguard the Well-Being of Youth with Behavioral and Emotional Challenges*. In this document, the GAO identifies problems with current regulations: "weakness in current federal-state regulatory structure have failed to safeguard the civil rights and well-being of some of the nation's most vulnerable youth, and we discuss the implications of some options for action that states, federal agencies, and Congress may consider in any restructure effort" (Government Accounting Office, 2008, p. 5). The GAO recommended a series of actions to address maltreatment and other threats to teens in residential treatment such as greater federal oversight of state accountability of youth in treatment and on-site visits to states (p. 39-40).

The outcome of the investigation and report was a bill sponsored by Congressman George Miller titled "H.R. 6358: Stop Child Abuse for Teens in Residential Treatment Act of 2008." The bill calls for the U.S. Department of Health and Human Services to federally regulate the wilderness therapy field as well as any public or private organization that provides substance abuse or mental health residential services to youth. This bill passed the House in 2008 but did not go to the Senate. (Congressman Miller would continue this legislative pressure, reintroducing the same or extremely similar bills calling for federal oversight, each Congress through 2015; Rep. Miller announced he will retire in 2016. (The bill was reintroduced to Committee in July 2015 by Rep. Schiff as H.R. 3060 but GovTrack reports no further action.).

2008: A Five-Year Follow-Up of a Survey of North American Outdoor Behavioral Healthcare Programs

Shortly after the GAO report was published, three researchers: Keith Russell, H. Lee Gillis, and T. Grant Lewis (2008), published a journal article titled "A Five-Year Follow-Up of a Survey of North American Outdoor Behavioral Healthcare Programs." This article highlights current practices in the field by surveying 65 programs (out of 102 requests) that fit an updated definition of an Outdoor Behavioral Healthcare. The article cites that the majority of outdoor behavioral healthcare programs follow an expedition format (either mountaineering or primitive skills based), are licensed by their state, and half of the programs are also accredited by a national organization. The "industry" of wilderness programs has actively updated what was previously referred to loosely as "wilderness therapy" into a more restrictive, objective definition: "outdoor behavioral healthcare (OBH) refers to programs that subscribe to a multimodal treatment model within the context of wilderness environments and backcountry travel to facilitate progress toward individualized treatment goals. The approach incorporates the use of evidenced-based clinical practices including client assessment, individual and group psychotherapy conducted by independently licensed clinicians, and the development of individual treatment and aftercare plans" (p. 62). This updated definition, which adds "independently licensed clinicians," reflects the current clinical emphasis of wilderness therapy programs.

2012: Publication of *Adventure Therapy: Theory, Research, and Practice*

In 2012, Mike Gass, Ph.D., from University of New Hampshire, Lee Gillis, Ph.D., from Georgia College, and Keith Russell, Ph.D., from Western Washington University, co-authored *Adventure Therapy: Theory, Research, and Practice*. This book is the most up to date academic text related to adventure and wilderness therapy practices. It covers a wide range of topics including ethics, competencies, assessment, and recent research tracks into wilderness therapy efficacy. It includes a chapter on the history of the field written by this author. In this book, adventure therapy is defined as "the prescriptive use of adventure experiences provided by mental health professionals, often conducted in natural setting that kinesthetically engage clients on cognitive, affective, and behavioral levels" (p. 1). While there remains some active dialogue about "adventure therapy" vs. "wilderness therapy," both the *Adventure Therapy* book and OBHC use nearly identical definitions for the experience, and differ mainly on required time in the natural setting.

2015: Wilderness and Adventure Therapy in Higher Education

With the growth in both the fields of wilderness and adventure therapy, there been a subsequent rise in graduate and undergraduate programs specializing to meet this growing field. As of 2015, there are three distinct graduate programs which all provide specialization for students. Prescott College offers a Masters in Arts (MA) program with a concentration in Adventure Based Counseling (Prescott.edu), Naropa University offers a Masters in Transpersonal Counseling (MA) with a Wilderness Therapy Concentration (http://www.naropa.edu), and most recently the University of New Hampshire offers a Dual Master Degree Program in Social Work (MSW) and Outdoor Education (MS) (http://chhs.unh.edu). These programs are from two to three years in length and students in all programs are required to participate in a specialized internship in a wilderness or adventure therapy setting. Unity College in Unity, Maine offers the only Bachelors Degree in Adventure Therapy (http://www.unity.edu). Faculty in all programs have relationships with both the OBH Council as well as AEE and are active leaders in the fields of adventure and wilderness therapy.

Summary

This section affirms psychiatrist Elton McNeil's 1957 prediction (cited on page 4 of this book) that "trained professionals" (p.23) would become more involved in wilderness therapy field and the field would expand. Yet McNeil's (1957) encouragement of research to "answer to the question of the effectiveness of therapeutic efforts" (p. 10) in wilderness settings is still in process. According to Russell (2007), "despite positive steps in identifying and improving best practices" in wilderness therapy, there is still a "paucity of research and evaluation" (p. 8) on practice and outcome yet the research is building (see Research Bibliography in Appendix). The current clinical emphasis in the field is very different from some of the early influences on the field that will be explored more in the next section.

This section chronicled some of the numerous individuals, models, organizations, books, and articles that influenced the emergence and long evolution of the field of wilderness therapy. This chapter primarily used documents as reference for the literature review and therefore, it should not be considered a complete history, due to the fact that much of the early history of the wilderness therapy field has not appeared in written form. What has been written in this history of the field included some documented controversies related to deaths and abuse but should not be seen as all-encompassing.

In chronicling the development of wilderness therapy in this section, several organizations emerged as the first to integrate new populations or practices into the field.

The first summer camp for psychologically challenged youth was founded in 1922 at Camp Ramapo in upstate New York. The first long-term residential wilderness camp for troubled youth, specifically, and the originator of the model that remained relevant and effective for the following 70 years, opened in 1946 at The Dallas Salesmanship Club Camp in Texas, integrating the first multi-day wilderness trips with troubled youth. The Outward Bound USA organization, founded in 1962, should be seen as the first to utilize a mountaineering style of wilderness therapy, as well as adding the solos, "marathons" and Final Expeditions where the students self-directed the entire concluding experience. And, Outward Bound USA developed or inspired numerous outdoor organizations for psychologically challenged youth. The BYU 480 program, started in 1968, should be seen as the first to utilize and popularize a primitive skills model to wilderness therapy and start the expansion of this model in the West.

The histories and influence of the Dallas Salesmanship Club Camp and Outward Bound USA on wilderness therapy are well documented by authors like Davis-Berman, Berman and Gass to name a few. The primitive skills school of wilderness therapy at BYU 480 and the primitive skills model that emerged from it has more recently been documented by White (2011). What until now was an oral history of outdoor behavioral healthcare programs in existence toay buntil now was an oral history of outdoor behavioral healthcare programs in existence today becomes the next section of this book.

Part II

Narratives from Present Day Programs

"When an old person dies it is like a library burns."

– Alex Hayley

THIS SECTION PRESENTS NARRATIVE HISTORIES from twenty-three wilderness therapy programs as well the Wilderness Therapy Symposium (WTS), Outdoor Behavioral Healthcare Council (OBH Council), and the Outdoor Behavioral Research Cooperative (OBHRC). The majority of the programs in this section are members of the Outdoor Behavioral Health Council (OBH). Also included are programs that could be members of OBH in the future or have been so in the past. It does not include programs that are closed. It also does not include all programs in the world as that would expand this book to several volumes. For those that I have missed I apologize. Some of the programs are for-profit and others are not. Some are in the United States and others in Canada. Some are reimbursed by their State entities, others by insurance, and others by parents. Three things that unite all of the programs are they fit the definition of an Outdoor Behavioral Healthcare Program, they are currently operating, and that they were willing to contribute by writing a chapter for this fundraising book.

This section began in the fall of 2014 when twenty-six invitations were sent to programs asking them to contribute their stories to this fundraising book. Twenty-six provided a chapter. The invitation requested a 4 to 5 page narrative account of the origins of the program that informed the reader of who were the founders, what were the influences that shaped the development of the programs, and what are the current operations of the program. What came back are stories as varied as ways to climb a bald peak. The stories reveal differences yet all reveal the similarities of helping people via the outdoors.

These accounts are narratives from the programs and any issue with the account should be brought directly to the author of the chapter. The accuracy of each story has not been validated by the main author and should be viewed as a narrative from the story tellers' perspective.

The chapters are placed in chronological order based on starting date. The reader should take time reading this section to get the sense of each program and how its story is told in order to get a sense of how the program evolved. Each program brings something unique to the field. Readers are encouraged to literally be in the outdoors or to picture themselves outside, perhaps around a campfire, while reading these stories from the field.

Chapter 3

1971: Project D.A.R.E. – Wendigo Lake

Steve Glass

http://wendigolake.com

STEEPED IN BUSH CRAFT AND WILDERNESS SURVIVAL through his boyhood involvement with the Australian Boy Scouts, Bob Davies had also been ocean sailing since the age of seven. Arriving in Canada as a young man, Bob was hired by the Ontario Ministry of Correctional Services to serve as a youth corrections worker. Davies soon built a reputation within the Ministry's senior management for developing and leading outdoor adventure camping programs which were viewed as having a very positive impact on the participants. On November 18, 1968, 33-year-old Bob Davies, who was now Camp Director at the Sprucedale Training School, submitted a brief proposal to his superiors to create a permanent camp to provide therapeutic adventure programming to adolescent multiple recidivists. In April, 1971, Project D.A.R.E. (Development through Adventure, Responsibility and Education) was launched at Portage Lake.

Project D.A.R.E.'s 84-day program was divided into three 28-day phases: the first phase focused on education and skill development, the second phase was bush camp service learning where those skills were applied, and the third phase of 'Outward Venture' culminated the experience with a full wilderness expedition.

Staff and students dressed the same and did everything together as co-participants.

On May 8, 1972 a second camp was opened on Wendigo Lake, near Algonquin Provincial Park, intended to serve younger first-time offenders.

A year later that program moved into a near-by purpose-built campus at Loxton Lake. In April 1976, the two Project D.A.R.E. programs were merged at the Loxton Lake campus where it has operated continuously ever since.

Bob Davies believed sailing would be a valuable addition to the Project D.A.R.E. program and a twenty-seven-foot Naval Whaler (open boat) was acquired in 1973. The S.V. Boomerang sailed up the St. Lawrence and through the Great Lakes over twenty-seven days, crewed by Bob Davies and nine of his staff who were "exposed to almost every conceivable type of weather and water conditions…to make sure all staff who would venture out with D.A.R.E. students on Georgian Bay were well trained and fully experienced in all aspects of boatmanship" (Davies, B.; 1973). Bob soon also introduced an equine component into the Portage Lake program with the addition of horses acquired from the Royal Canadian Mounted Police. Project D.A.R.E. rose to national prominence and was featured in the prime time TV show called *This Land* by the Canadian Broadcasting Corporation, entitled 'From Out of the Wilderness'. Frustrated at how Project D.A.R.E.'s implementation was drifting from his vision, Bob Davies wrote a three and a half page memo to all staff entitled "General Philosophy and Objectives of Project D.A.R.E." in which he outlines the program's core principles (Davies, B. 1975). Learning is by example, and staff will exemplify and perform every task and attitude asked of a student. All members of the group (staff and students) are responsible for and accountable to the group with staff leadership. Programming will offer a progression of challenge and skill development, promote the program motto to "Seek Your Horizon," reveal the metaphysical realm of life as more important than the physical realm, respect the student's dignity, social, physical and emotional needs, and require staff to present as caring persons and not as strict authoritarian figures. His memo concludes with the following:

> The 'Statement of Objectives' is the whole foundation
> D.A.R.E. was based upon. Each person employed at
> D.A.R.E. should be aware of the objectives and strive towards
> attaining these goals with the students and their fellow staff.
> It is easy to lose sight of these objectives once we become
> enmeshed in the everyday struggle for our own survival.
> Some of you may say that these objectives are too idealistic. If

that is the case, I would suggest that you seek lesser horizons which are not so demanding in some other type of institution of life.

Unfortunately, a study comparing the subsequent delinquent behavior and work/school involvement of graduates from the Portage Lake Project D.A.R.E. program with that of youth placed in traditional training schools found that participants in the D.A.R.E. program "… did not do as well as was expected after graduation" (Birkenmayer A., Polonoski M.; 1976, p.13) and these findings had a significant impact on both the future operations and government support for the program. As Bob Davies moved on to his next adventure, his successors over the next four decades repeatedly modified the program design to achieve greater individualized programming matched to students' risks and needs, and pursued program manualization and tracking of outcomes to improve the program. Project D.A.R.E. sought to innovate and respond to the changing needs of Ontario's at-risk and behaviorally-challenging youth, driven by the almost constant fear that some remote government decision would kill the program and a fierce pride and conviction that 'a bad day at Project D.A.R.E. is better than a great day at a traditional custody facility'. The fear of closure was not misplaced – several times over the years formal plans have been created to close Project D.A.R.E., each time forestalled by forceful advocacy from the vast community of people whose lives have been positively impacted – program participants, past staff, parents, probation officers, judges, civil servants and influential political figures. Throughout the decades, the universally acknowledged core strength of Project D.A.R.E. has been its success in attracting staff, particularly Instructors, who have demonstrated skillful enthusiasm and concern for giving students their very best and building strong therapeutic relationships.

In 1992, Dr. Adam Lodzinski, retained by the government to conduct an exhaustive literature review and develop a resource-book for evidence-informed programming across Ontario's entire youth justice system, agreed to undertake an outcomes study of Project D.A.R.E. graduates. His conclusion was that, "In sum, the available evidence suggests DARE's secure custody recidivism rate compares favorably… (and)…it is clear that DARE's environment sustains therapeutically meaningful activities that no other facility in this province can offer." (Lodzinski, A.; 1992).

In 1996 Stephen Glass arrived as the new Administrator of Project D.A.R.E., on what was supposed to be a six-month developmental assignment. Glass soon recognized in the Project D.A.R.E. staff an intense sense of commitment to Project D.A.R.E.'s ideals and a palpable sense of community – and the developmental opportunity was transformed into a sense of vocation to protect and develop Project D.A.R.E. to its full potential. In 1998 the government announced its intention to privatize Project D.A.R.E. Glass incorporated Wendigo Lake Expeditions and submitted the successful proposal to operate Project D.A.R.E. as of July 2000.

Wendigo Lake Expeditions retained Dr. Keith Russell to conduct an outcomes study (2002), became accredited by the Association for Experiential Education (2003), became a member of the Outdoor Behavioral Healthcare Council (2003), launched a new adventure therapy program for non-adjudicated youth (2003) and commenced employing masters-level therapists (2005). Wendigo Lake Expeditions continues to operate the Project D.A.R.E. open custody therapeutic adventure program as well as a small-group adventure therapy residential treatment program designed to support family permanency under Glass's leadership.

Chapter 4

1976: ENVIROS

Bev Oldham

http://www.enviros.org

DURING THE FALL AND WINTER OF 1976 THE FIRST group of Enviros Youth Workers and volunteers, along with eight youth, ventured into the eastern slopes of the Rocky Mountains near Banff National Park. This group was a mixed gender collection of young people all of whom were experiencing some life challenges either in the form of substance abuse, conflict with the law, grief and loss, trauma and or family conflict and discord. This outing was not merely a "recreational outing" rather, it was an exercise in self-discipline and personal growth lasting eight months. While living in tents and completing school on-site with distance learning modules, the youth persevered and succeeded in building the first Enviros Wilderness facility, Enviros Base Camp. This success founded the legacy of experiential learning, which has become the Enviros trademark in child, youth, adult and family services.

Today, Enviros is a charitable, non-profit community of people committed to enhancing the quality of family life in Alberta by offering a variety of experiential-based programs to assist children, youth, adults and families in learning and developing skills that foster independence. Since our early beginnings Enviros has expanded to address a broad range of societal needs, including programs for: young offenders, foster care, FASD, Youth Transition to Adulthood, group and intensive treatment programs, respite care connections, High-Fidelity Wrap Around services as well as our Base Camp and Shunda Creek addiction treatment programs. Enviros continues to utilize the outdoors as a therapeutic strategy within a majority of our programs, while working with the young person, their families and their community. Base Camp and Shunda Creek use adventure therapy as one of their key treatment modalities.

Base Camp

Enviros Base Camp is a wilderness based residential treatment center for youth and families in Alberta struggling with addiction issues. It is a 90-day, 10-bed program that is open to both males and females ages 12-18. The facility is located in the remote Ghost Forest northwest of Calgary and is an off-grid facility accessible via a rough logging road. The program, in collaboration with Alberta Health Services, addresses substance abuse issues that are better served through residential treatment and support in a wilderness setting that uses adventure therapy and wilderness therapeutically. The program is family based, with a commitment to change being made with the family unit. Base Camp supports extensive family involvement and strikes a balance between addiction treatment, building on family strengths, traditional schooling, outdoor education and community experiences. The aim is to support persons served and their families in creating lasting, positive change.

The program is designed to address individual client needs in a group milieu. Much of the program is delivered by Youth and Family Support Workers with the oversight of shift supervisors and family therapists. The program is built around the "Circle of Courage," primarily the needs that clients have with regards to belonging, mastery, independence and generosity. Clients work with staff to develop "personal plans" that guide the work they're doing individually in treatment. Clients also engage in milieu treatment, groups (psycho-educational, process and ceremonial), wilderness trips, traditional schooling and family therapy, which are guided by addressing common needs that include; improving emotional regulation, improving physical health, strengthening executive function, cultivating communication skills, improving relationships, building self-efficacy and planning for transition.

There are a few practices that the program considers fundamental to delivering best-practice treatment opportunities, which include Non-Violent Communication, Experiential and Wilderness/Adventure Therapy, Motivational Interviewing, Mindfulness Based Stress Reduction and Group Facilitation/Processing. These practices are embedded in all aspects of the program and provide a foundation for highly individualized treatment processes. The program is also utilizing a "feedback informed treatment" process where client's reported outcomes (through a variety of instruments and questionnaires) are directly returned to the frontline staff in a weekly format to serve as both progress monitoring and information for clients to create personal plans. Base Camp is currently in year one of a "Project to Explore Treatment Outcomes," a research and evaluation project undertaken by our co-principal investigators Keith C. Russell, Ph.D Western Washington University and H.L. (Lee) Gillis, Ph.D. Georgia College & State University.

Shunda Creek

Shunda Creek provides a 10-bed residential addiction treatment program for young adult males between the ages of 18-24 and their families by providing intensive adventure based wilderness programming. Shunda Creek is located 3 hours NW of Calgary, Alberta situated along the eastern slopes of the Alberta Rockies. The program was developed in response to the growing gang involvement of young adult males the same population who identified that the standard government treatment facilities were not meeting their particular treatment needs. In collaboration with Alberta Health Services Shunda Creek addresses substance abuse issues within a wilderness setting that better meets the treatment needs of a young adult male population. The program is family based, with a commitment to change being made with the family unit. Shunda Creek supports extensive family involvement and in collaboration with our partner Alberta Health Services Addiction and Mental Health through the provision of quarterly family based weekend treatment retreats. Family members come out to Shunda Creek to participate in group and individual work as well as to explore their relationships with one another through the use of experiential activities. Shunda Creek uses evidence supported treatment that puts the relationship between the client and the therapist and the supporting staff at the center of the healing process. We are continually building a community and a culture of mindfulness, shared journey, compassionate inquiry, right use of power, and intentionality. It is an ongoing daily process seeking towards integrity where everything fits together, every moment of every day.

Shunda Creek is an open enrollment 90-day psycho-educationally based residential adventure therapy model. The treatment approach uses a variety of different treatment modalities fusing Experiential Learning, Adventure Therapy, Motivational Interviewing, Cognitive Behavioral Treatment, social skills training, behavioral contracting, mindfulness practice, yoga and core tenets of group therapy facilitated by the treatment team. In the Shunda Creek model, adventure therapy is the primary tool used to enhance a more traditional addictions treatment model and is not seen as adjunct or tangential. Each client develops an individual treatment plan in consultation with the lead clinician that includes goals, action plans, and additional measurable indicators that provide support for progress being made on the treatment plan. There are daily group meetings, periodic weekly or drop-in visits with the lead clinician and daily brief teachable moments by the staff and clients through shared experience and daily living. The therapeutic relationship, driven by the client, to support the client's needs, with the lead clinician, staff and peers forms the core of the treatment model being delivered by Shunda Creek. Staff believes strongly that the treatment process at Shunda Creek is a shared journey that is co-created with the client. As staff they must meet the client where they are at with regards to their addictions and desire to change. Shunda Creek is currently in year four of a *Project to Explore Treatment Outcomes*. As well, we have recently received two year funding to conduct the *Shunda Creek Alumni Evauolation Project*. Our co-principal investigators for both research projects are Keith C. Russell, Ph.D Western Washington University and H.L. (Lee) Gillis, Ph.D. Georgia College & State University

Shunda Creek does not consider clients who complete their 12 weeks of treatment as graduates. Rather they are passing into the next phase in their journey of addiction recovery. When a client has completed their 12 weeks we recognize the event as a passage. Clients create a "passage" trip in week 10 that they believe best reflects their growth in treatment and sets an intention for the next phase of their recovery. These passage trips may include new clients coming in to treatment as a way for the outgoing clients to share their experience in treatment. We have a ceremony that celebrates the client work in treatment prior to them leaving Shunda

Creek. Shunda Creek is also funded to provide Alumni outreach and support to those clients who have *passaged* from the Shunda Creek program and have returned to live in their communities. Shunda Creek has provided follow-up/outreach support to former clients for the past three years.

Chapter 5

1984: Brief History of Marimed Foundation

Matt Claybaugh

http://marimed.org

Honolulu-based Marimed Foundation (from "maritime medicine") was established in 1984 by Harvard-educated lawyer and ship captain David Higgins and his Ob/Gyn wife, Dr. Lonny Higgins. Its initial mission was to support the development of outer island dispensaries in the Republic of the Marshall Islands ("RMI") using a specially-designed tall ship, staffed by medical professional volunteers and RMI Ministry of Health staff, making regular training and logistical support "rounds" throughout the remote atolls where there were no airstrips. From 1984 through 1987, Dr. Higgins took volunteers to the outer atolls using copra freighters and chartered fishing boats for transportation while her husband raised funds for the design and building of the ship and recruited board members for the Foundation. Initial board members included Dr. Bill Walsh, founder of Project Hope, Gilbert Grosvenor, President of The National Geographic Society, and Dr. Jonas Salk of the Salk Institute.

The Foundation's tall ship, designed by New Zealand's Ted Ewbank and named *Tole Mour* ("gift of life and health") by the school children of the Marshall Islands, was commissioned in Seattle in 1988. A steel, 156-foot, three-masted, square topsail schooner, *Tole Mour* had accommodations for 26 crew and staff, and contained lab and clinic space, an x-ray room, and a cytology lab. In all, the *Tole Mour* served 50 small communities on a dozen atolls from 1988 to 1992. In 1990, a service-learning program for teens from both Hawaii and the RMI was added, with the youth supporting the traveling medical teams ashore and engaging in service-learning and week-long, intra-atoll "survival" exercises using Pete Kalajian dories.

By 1991, the RMI's budget for its outer island dispensary system had tripled, airstrips had been built on a number of remote atolls, and the RMI Ministry of Health had acquired a vessel of its own able to make health training rounds. Moreover, as planned, *Tole Mour's* ex-patriot medical director, nursing staff, dental team, and deckhands had all been replaced by their Marshallese counterparts. At the same time in Hawaii, the need for innovative approaches to the challenges of treating and educating Hawaii youth with behavioral challenges was reaching crisis proportions. In 1992, Marimed returned *Tole Mour* to Hawaii and, building on its service learning program experience, began providing behavioral health care for special needs Hawaii youth. To assist in this transformation, the organization turned to experts in wilderness therapy, youth corrections, cross-cultural and ship-based programs, including Peter Willauer (Hurricane Island and Thompson Island Outward Bound), Dr. Manu Meyer (University of Hawaii), Candi Kane (Summit Achievement), and Lorraine Robinson (Ka Hale Ho'ala Hou No Na Wahine). Program design was also influenced by site visits to the Fulton Foundation in Assens, Denmark. With the help of Capt. Wallace Stark and Rafe Parker of Sea Education Association, *Tole Mour* was renovated to provide accommodations for 49 and to meet Coast Guard requirements for licensure as a USCG Sailing School Vessel.

In 1993, Marimed's President and CEO, Dr. Matt Claybaugh, joined as a program director and spearheaded a two-year joint venture with Arizona-based VisionQuest. This was a ship-based, rolling admissions program for 28 court-referred youth from several states, including Hawaii. This program took *Tole Mour* and her court-referred youth crew from Hawaii through the Panama Canal, along the eastern seaboard, and up the St. Lawrence to Erie, Pennsylvania, and back. Its success was due in large part to the efforts of Chris Mays of Point School Puerto Rico (then with VisionQuest).

In 2000, Marimed sold *Tole Mour* to Guided Discoveries and acquired its current ship, Makani Olu, a 96-foot, steel three-masted staysail schooner with accommodations for 20. The sale of *Tole Mour* also allowed Marimed to purchase community-based homes to house the "cadets" when onshore. One of the early challenges Marimed faced once committing fully to serving high-risk adolescents was economies of scale. *Tole Mour* needed to house 16-20 cadets at a time to remain a viable platform for therapy. By downsizing the ship and its related expenses and moving the cadets to shore-side facilities with a maximum capacity of 8 cadets each, Marimed was better able to manage challenging behaviors and to more fully individualize therapy. Cadets could now participate in voyages as a "house-community," and staff could focus on the needs of 8 rather than 20 while at sea.

While voyaging aboard tall ships and experientially educating cadets have been cornerstones of Marimed's adolescent programs since 1990, where personal growth and role transformation were identified as ideal outcomes for cadets, identifying the model as wilderness therapy was still a ways off.

Kailana (Calm Seas), Marimed's oldest adolescent behavioral healthcare program (est. 1993), began as a residential treatment program that incorporated boat building and daily ocean-based activities (rowing, sailing, and Hawaiian canoe paddling) with individual and group therapy sessions. The Kailana model, still in practice, became the template for how Marimed blends western therapeutic notions and practices (often called the "medical model"), outdoor adventure programming, and culturally aligned norms and traditions into one hybridized treatment model well suited for the Hawaii adolescent population.

After years at Marimed, Dr. Claybaugh tried to capture aspects of this multidisciplinary culturally-rooted model of education, growth and transformation and its relationship to ocean voyaging in his dissertation, "The Sea Change in American Sea Narratives: An Experiential Perspective," (1998). The process of collecting theories from across disciplines and sharing them with staff members – from the likes of John Dewey and Howard Gardner, to Richard Kimball, John Hendee, and Michael Brown, combined with a sea narrative tradition of personal change at sea found in the likes of Richard Henry Dana Jr. and Robin Lee Graham – encouraged the Kailana treatment model to take shape and build a strong theoretical foundation for what we now call Ocean-based wilderness therapy.

In 2014, Marimed was the first non-land-based program accepted into the Outdoor Behavioral Healthcare Council, and is pursuing the accreditation.

Responding to community need in the years following the creation of Kailana, Marimed has operated several independent programs or partnered with other agencies to provide services to male and female youth, families and adults. Marimed has been nationally accredited for behavioral health and substance abuse treatment since 2000. All the programs utilize the foundation of the Kailana model and experiential-based learning for change. As the Ocean-based wilderness therapy model evolved and solidified, Dr. Claybaugh pushed for outcomes studies of the effectiveness of the Kailana model. Published outcome studies showing program effectiveness include: *Outcome Evaluation Findings of a Hawaiian Culture-Based Adolescent Substance Abuse Treatment Program,* Psychological Services 2009, Catalyst Group, LLC, and *Impact of Culturally Relevant Residential Treatment Program on Post-Discharge Outcomes for Hawaii Youth,* published in the Journal of Therapeutic Schools and Programs 2010, University of New Hampshire.

Through the years Marimed has developed a distinct competency and is considered a premier provider of experiential learning services in the Pacific. Today, Marimed operates several residential, after-school, and short-term community-chartered experiential programs, as well as vocational programs. While each of these programs is distinct, at their core is the Kailana model and the real-life, hands-on challenge and change experiences that occur during Ocean-based wilderness therapy and voyaging aboard *Makani Olu.*

Chapter 6

1987: Anasazi Foundation

Ezekiel Sanchez (Good Buffalo Eagle)

http://www.anasazi.org

IN 1965, MY FIRST YEAR AT BRIGHAM YOUNG UNIVERSITY (BYU), I flunked out because I had not really been prepared for college life. Since I had received an art scholarship, I attended faithfully my art classes but was not ready for studying in other classes. I went back home and was hired by the Union Pacific Railroad in Las Vegas, Nevada, to be part of the crew as a gandy dancer (railroad worker). So I was back to hard labor in the hot sun, but I did not tell my family I had flunked out. Every day after work my brothers and sisters would ask me about university life. The more I related the campus experiences, the more my heart wanted to be back to BYU.

So one night, I decided I was not going to drink or eat until I found a way back to BYU. When I arrived that morning to work, the crew boss announced he had received a call for us to remove all the railroad ties and steel railings and set new ones in. For a moment, I thought maybe this is not a time to go without food and water, but I had made up my mind. When I got home after not eating or drinking water, my mother met me at the door. My mother took one look at me and said, "Are you okay, son?" I told her I was okay. She then said, "You make sure you eat tonight because I prepared your favorite food," and as she walked away into the dark hallway, she said, "By the way, there's a letter for you on the kitchen table."

1968: BYU 480 Survival

I had never received a letter in my entire life – maybe it was because I had never written one. The return address said Brigham Young University. I tore the letter open, and it read something like this: "Dear academic dropout, my name is Larry D. Olsen. The university has asked me to conduct an experimental program out in the wilderness. If you'd like to be a guinea pig and go with me, and if you live through the experience, you'll be admitted back on probation to the university."

Now, a lot of people might call that coincidence. But I had gone without food and water, pleading with the heavens to help me find a way to get back to the university. I felt that letter was an answer to my pleadings. I was going back to BYU.

Once on the campus, I went looking for Larry D. Olsen and finally found his office. Larry's desk was against the wall, so his back was to the door. I asked, "Are you Larry D. Olsen?" He said, "Yes, I am he. Sit down; I'll be done in a minute." Soon Larry turned around, and the first thing I noticed was his glasses, which resembled the bottom of Coca-Cola bottles. I asked in disbelief, "Are you the Larry Olsen that's going to take us out on the trail?" He said, "Yes, I am he." I thought to myself, "Oh, he's going to kill us," and I made a judgment of Larry. Later I rescinded that judgment, because when we were in the field, he was like Super Survivor Man.

When we went out on the first trip, there was a nurse that the university sent with Larry by the name of Doris Jackson. She was in her late 60's. She couldn't keep up, and when she got sick on the second day, Larry sent her out. By the third day, Larry snuck into my camp and pulled me to one side. He told me of the things he'd recognized I already knew; about edibles and this and that. He told me what had happened to Doris Jackson, and he said, "I need you to help me develop this program." The first night I said "no" because I promised my family I would finish my studies at BYU. After a night of sleep I changed my mind to help Larry. That started a good partnership and adventure unlike anything else I have experienced in my life.

If I had any word to use to describe the trail experiences starting with the first BYU walking, from my perspective, it would be "majestic." Why? Because it has really affected my heart and my life – the way I think and act. By the time I finished that course, I knew I was someone special. I knew I was here for a purpose. What purpose it was, I knew not. I worked with Larry for numerous years at BYU 480 and on other courses but would leave to do other projects, and 19 years later Larry approached me again while I was working at the Missionary Training Center on campus.

Anasazi

Larry came to me in 1987 and said we should start a program based on our early principles and work at BYU. I had a good job at the Missionary Training Center, so I again went without food and water to find my way back to BYU. I also invited my family to go without food and water to know whether or not to go with Larry. At the end of fasting for 24 hours, I asked my family, how they felt about Larry's request. The four oldest children who participated said we were supposed to go with Larry. And my wife, Pauline, who is never prone to make any hasty decisions, also said, "I feel we should join Larry."

That night, I slept uneasily because my children were asking, "Dad, what did you tell Larry?" Somewhere in the morning I had a dream, and I saw a multitude of children lined up, coming toward me, some of them hugging me and thanking me for the small part I played in their lives. I woke up and I told my wife, "We're going with Larry."

What I am doing today with Anasazi Foundation is not what I planned to do with my life. But I was sent, and because the Creator sent me, I'm here. I know it's a sacred time for me to be here. Once I had that dream, I didn't doubt anymore. I knew we'd find a way to feed and clothe my family, because after all, we're survivalists, right?

In 1994, five years after we started Anasazi, Larry left to Buhl, Idaho, to manage the Miracle Hot Springs he had inherited from his dad. But by then Anasazi had already become a non-profit, and we had a great team with Mike Merchant, Sterling Tanner, and L. Paul Newman, as well as my family and several other good people who were part of the Anasazi Team.

I will speak briefly about the Anasazi Way philosophy. Our philosophy states that all the two-legged beings have a seed of greatness with potential to succeed. We call the children Young Walkers, because they are young and they are doing a walking. We teach the Young Walkers that the Creator has given us a Gift of Choice. This gift of choice gives us the power to choose how to walk in life. There are two ways one can walk in life. We choose to walk forward or to walk backward, and with every step we take forward or backward, we're accountable. And because we are accountable, there are consequences. Sometimes they come immediately; at other times the consequences are delayed. The Anasazi Way principles teach that all of us are responsible for our own choices.

Once the children realize they have the power to choose, they will choose knowingly. They cannot say "The devil made me do it or peer pressure made me do it, therefore it's not my fault." They now know they have the Gift of Choice to choose to walk away from peer pressure, from drugs, from anger, etc. It's a beautiful way of painting hope in their hearts and minds. The children love the Anasazi Way because it's a simple way.

So let me repeat what I just shared with you, as if you were a Young Walker. You have a Seed of Greatness. You're a Sacred Being. And you have a gift given by the Creator, called the Gift of Choice. Along with the Gift of Choice, you were born knowing right from wrong. That's called conscience. And there are two ways you can walk, according to the Navajo language. Walking forward is making good choices and walking backward is making wrong choices. So, life is walking – a journey in which we choose according to the heart. If your heart's at war, which way will you walk? If your heart's at peace, which way will you walk?

The Anasazi Way is not geared to change behavior but to change the heart. We don't have steps or levels. We're striving to touch the heart because, if we can touch the heart, the Young Walker will change his/her behavior, and then they own the change.

That is quite a mouthful, isn't it? I'm here with you today, known not only as Ezekiel, but also as Good Buffalo Eagle. I went to BYU to be an artist, but changed my major to Youth Leadership because of what Larry and I were doing. And as a Founder of Anasazi Foundation, I am an artist of a different kind. Today I paint in children's hearts a better picture of themselves.

I am Good Buffalo Eagle, and I have spoken.

Chapter 7

1992: Omni Youth Services – Journey

Sean Hoyer and John Conway

http://www.omniyouth.org/programs-services/adventure-therapy-services

Omni Youth Services' Journey: Skills for life adventure therapy program was influenced by many individuals and it could be argued that the program is as old as the agency itself, starting in 1972. However, the program as is experienced today was most notably influenced by three individuals: Mark Wall, Sean Hoyer and John Conway.

Mark was exposed to the impact of a wilderness setting at a very early age. His father ran a summer camp for juvenile offenders in Lake of the Woods, Ontario and he was immediately struck by the powerful effect moving some youth out of their home environments had. In his early adult years, Mark and his father worked with adolescent male offenders who were incarcerated for 30, 60 or 90 days. They did 1 to 14 day trips year round in one of the most beautiful areas of North America. The groups had tens of thousands of miles of pristine wilderness all to themselves. The staff ate, slept, worked and explored with the residents. This experience provided an alternative way for the juvenile offenders to see themselves and experience ongoing mastery, self-control, and community.

In 1990, after grad school, Mark applied to OMNI Youth Services. OMNI had just started a therapeutic adventure program and Mark was able to join in early, bring his existing "hard" skills, while growing his therapeutic "soft" skills. The evolution of the program was invigorating, challenging and creative.

Sean Hoyer "discovered" wilderness therapy as a 15 year old on a 10-day canoe trip in the Quetico Wilderness in Canada. During that experience, Sean realized that he wanted a career that used the outdoors to assist people make changes – just as he had experienced in his youth and young adult years. He set about developing the knowledge and skills to support what he felt were the position attributes of a career he did not know the name of. He developed leadership and responsibility, camp craft and wilderness travel, safety and judgment, the ability to speak well and the capacity to listen even better. Along the way, Sean sought the advice of mentors that each reflected that they saw no job in the mix of these seemingly disparate skill sets, adding that maybe he could do some of the camping "stuff" as a hobby after he got a real job. In 1996, Sean happened into a job fair at his grad school with a copy of a resume in his back pocket. After 20 minutes of wandering past a sea of potential careers, he was drawn in by a program that was looking for what they themselves thought was an unrealistic combination of education, skills, experience, and aptitude. Instead, this was a perfect match for his decade of investment – combined under the umbrella of wilderness therapy, his passion and pursuits had found a home.

John grew up car camping with his family and spent his early adolescent years outdoors with the Boy Scouts of America, learning camp craft and admiring leaders who were willing to take the time to not only teach skills, but to walk along an often tumultuous path, working through the physical, psychological and emotional struggles of young men. John received his bachelor's degree in psychology and then went to work at a psychiatric hospital working on the child and adolescent unit while working on his MSW. This particular psychiatric facility had an indoor climbing wall and an outdoor team's course – fairly progressive for the early 90's – and… did John become a climbing guide? While pursuing his clinical degree, John became aware of programs in the "West" that utilized outdoor environments and adventure to reach young people. But never did it occur that any such programs existed or could exist in the Midwest. Similar to Sean, while John was at a job fair at his graduate program in May, 1996, he was introduced to OMNI Youth Services and immediately joined the team.

In 1992 OMNI had separated out four positions from the counseling programs to go forward with a substance abuse team. Ron Heinsman, who had been at OMNI for about two years, was recruited by OMNI's then clinical Director, Jay Meyer (presently Executive Director) to lead an expedition with substance abuse clients. Ron provided the tactical leadership and implementation that developed it into our current meaningful modality, The Journey: Skills for Life program. With Ron's departure in 1995 to pursue a calling as a missionary, the program leadership shifted to Mark Wall, a licensed clinical counselor. With his extensive outdoor technical and wilderness leadership experience he, under the direction of Jay Meyer, provided a prototype of a staff member who could effortlessly combine clinical and technical skills to effect change in adolescents and families in the office or in the wilderness. A core team of six staff were developed and valuable time and resources were invested to improve the core competencies of the group. Effective team members were expected to excel in five areas: interpersonal, clinical, technical, wilderness, and safety/judgment. Mark advocated that an individual or team that was "out of balance" with regard to these skills spent too much time compensating and not enough time intervening.

Mark's departure in 2000 left the team with a few seasoned staff but a need to develop intentional structures to institutionalize the program beyond a particular person or shared memory. Sean was instrumental in developing policies and procedures, expanding Journey's experiential and adventure-based programming. Within 5 years, the Journey: Skills For Life program boasted a dozen highly trained staff, provided over 120 days of programming a year, attained CoA accreditation, and recognition by the Association for Experiential Education as the Organizational Member of the Year, in 2005. The Journey program continued to grow and branch out into new areas and collaborative relationships under the leadership of John Conway. We became members of the relatively young consortium of highly acclaimed wilderness programs known as the Outdoor Behavioral Healthcare Industry Cooperative. In fact, OMNI was only the second not-for-profit program (Anasazi being the first) to be invited to join. It was felt by the founding members of OBHIC that the infusion of OMNI's ideology and philosophy to provide Adventure Therapy services to families all along the socio-economic scale, as well as the unique "clinically-intensive" model would benefit the entire industry.

We continue to get the question of how a community based counseling agency in the suburbs of a major city, hundreds of miles away from the wilderness would consider developing a wilderness therapy program. All of the contemporary program models were East-coast programs based on a boarding school concept with frequent, short-duration adventures as part of a months-long residential stay. In contrast, the "west-coast" model was described as "stripping away" the old behaviors through expeditionary trips in remote locations resulting in youth developing skills to transfer back home when they returned after 21 or 56 days.

OMNI's model developed from necessity; a high concentration of families in the suburbs of Chicago could obviously benefit from an intense clinical experience that might jump start treatment, refocus counseling efforts, or serve as the "graduation" by demonstrating a consolidation of skills gained through successful engagement in outpatient work.

Our program model thrives from ready access to a pool of clients and year-round access to a variety of wilderness settings. This allows us to have clients repeat in the modality throughout the year to advance their clinical gains and never have to repeat a trip modality. The wilderness setting allowed us as therapists the opportunities to observe our young clients responding to their circumstances in real time, rather than coming to a therapy session and reporting verbally. We were able to intervene in real time in the shared setting. We then helped clients think through how to translate what they learned and experienced to similar situations back at home. Over time we also focused on integrating what was learned more intentionally into the therapy sessions with the therapists back in the office.

Chapter 8

1993: RedCliff Ascent Wilderness Program

Kumen Jones

http://www.redcliffascent.com

T HE REDCLIFF ASCENT (RCA) WILDERNESS program began operation in 1993. It was the fourth therapeutic treatment program for troubled youth organized and run by Dane Kay, Steve (Cub) Petersen, Scott Petersen, and Jim Salisbury.

History of RCA

Cub first became interested in the idea of treating troubled youth in the early 1980s while he was working with youth from the Utah State Division of Juvenile Justice System. Through his work there, he developed a strong orientation towards experiential treatment and the value of work opportunities in treatment. At about that same time, Cub hired Jim and Dane at the lock up facility where he worked, and it became clear immediately that they subscribed to the same operating philosophy as he did.

In 1989, Jim and Cub decided to strike out on their own and start their own program. They found a facility in Orem on Sandhill Road and renovated it. They then applied for and received a contract with the Division of Youth Corrections and enrolled their first student in October 1989.

When Jim and Cub opened the Orem group home, they hired Dane Kay to work the graveyard shift while he was studying for his Finance Degree at BYU's Marriot School of Management. It so happened that one of his friends and classmates there was Cub's brother Scott Petersen, who was studying Marketing.

Eventually, Dane approached Scott about joining the enterprise, because he felt that Scott's marketing degree would provide a critical contribution to the future success of the business. Scott did, in fact, join the company in January of 1990.

At that point, the company was reorganized and split evenly among the four partners. Each of them brought a unique piece to the puzzle, and each was deeply committed to the others personally and professionally. Although they did not realize it at the time, the guiding principles and practices they adopted at the outset of their partnership laid the foundation for their future success.

Between 1990 and 1993, the boys (as they are called by those who work with them) added the Individual Residential Treatment (IRT) proctor program and in 1993 the company won a contract with the State of Utah to provide an "innovative alternative to secure care." They were pursuing a strategy of horizontal integration along the treatment continuum. This led to the creation of the Ascent Country Residential (ACR) facility located in Mona, Utah (30 miles south of Provo). At the same time they started the RedCliff Ascent (RCA) wilderness program and coupled that with the residential treatment experience at Mona.

RedCliff's first office was in the Executive Director's mobile home. From there the headquarters were moved to a storage facility in St. George, Utah, then to an old post office building, then to a house in Beryl Junction, and finally the offices in Enterprise, Utah (about 40 miles west of Cedar City and 40 miles north of St. George) which RCA still calls home.

The opening of RedCliff Ascent became the springboard for the company's entrance into the private market. This completed its horizontal integration in the public sector as it had everything from wilderness treatment to residential treatment to foster or proctor care and outpatient services.

Program Philosophy and Why it is Unique

RedCliff's emphasis has always been in using the wilderness for both assessment *and* treatment. As Dane Kay explained, "Our philosophy has *always* been that the more experiential the treatment environment, the more likely we will find a way into the kid and foster change."

"What we use," added Jim Salisbury, "is a continuous flow model with a strong orientation towards being accomplishment based. The clinical model is based on providing a safe environment where we can disrupt the negative patterns that kids and families have become enmeshed in. We then use the wilderness environment and well trained and caring staff to help kids learn new skills and prepare them to transition into the world in a productive way."

"There is an emphasis on hard skills," Cub Observed, "as metaphorical learning opportunities for the kids as well as opportunities for observation and assessment by our clinicians and program staff.

"We also require concurrent treatment on the part of the family. We believe strongly that the strength of our program is in our people. We have been fortunate to have attracted and retained some of the best people in the industry and the maturity and treatment record of the program speaks to that longevity and loyalty."

Dane, Cub, Scott, and Jim have a unique perspective on their business, because they worked every position in the company for the first few years. They hired the therapists and were able to assess their effectiveness based on what the partners saw, heard and experienced with the students when the therapists were not around. It was here that they developed their treatment philosophy of balance between the clinical team and the residential/field staff. They came to understand that there must be a balanced team effort. Because of this, RedCliff Ascent has been able to develop an efficient business model, as well as an effective therapeutic program. As Scott Petersen explained, "This, we believe, is a truly unique feature of our approach to treating troubled teens. Additionally, because our operation and expansion have been funded entirely from within the company, we have never had to answer to a detached outside board of directors. These two features have allowed us to focus on the best way to fulfill our mission of treating troubled youth."

Chapter 9

1996: Outdoor Behavioral Healthcare Council

Gil Hallows

https://obhcouncil.com

DURING THE LATE 1980S AND EARLY 90S, A NUMBER of wilderness programs emerged based on the concept that taking at-risk youth out into the wilds for extended, group-oriented and simplified living expeditions could produce improved behavior, stronger sense of self, and the mitigation of many emotional and mental health issues. During this early period of program development, some programs failed to pay proper attention to such concerns as risk management and quality of therapeutic care. There occurred a series of unfortunate incidents, including several deaths, which resulted in the prevailing media coverage of the field of wilderness therapy being negative and critical.

With this atmosphere as the backdrop, a small group of visionary leaders from a handful of wilderness programs got together to test the premise that it would serve the interests of their students, their families and their individual businesses to pause competition and test if they could work together to establish basic standards around quality of care and managing risk.

In the early summer of 1996, representatives from Anasazi, Aspen Achievement Academy, Catherine Freer, Redcliff Ascent, and SUWS sat looking at each other around a table in Salt Lake City pondering the potential benefits of collaboration. Each attendee at this seminal gathering quickly came to see that the others were committed to doing good work and held strong convictions that wilderness therapy is a powerful and effective treatment modality. The mutual conclusion was that all could trust each other and all would benefit by working together to advance the field of wilderness therapy.

Through the next meetings, the group coined the term "outdoor behavioral healthcare" (OBH) to establish common language for the field. The OBH Council set about establishing a vision and identifying a mission. Like the mythical table of King Arthur's, every member organization was expected to contribute equally and to their abilities and so members agreed to work on the various detailed OBHC committees, and gather 3 times a year for Association-wide discussion and votes. Many of the possible agendas discussed gravitated into the broad areas of managing risk, delivering effective treatment, and measuring the effectiveness of what we were doing.

Very early on, it became clear that simply turning up the volume of our proclamations that wilderness therapy is effective was not sufficient. If we expected anyone to take our claims seriously, we needed substantiating research. OBHC's mission statement emerged from this intensive process, and continues to guide the OBH Council's initiatives to the present:

> The Outdoor Behavioral Healthcare Council is a
> community of leading outdoor behavioral healthcare
> programs working to advance the field through best practices,
> effective treatment, and evidence-based research.

Under the leadership of Rob Cooley, the first chair of OBHC, the group came to realize that conducting and supporting research was perhaps the single most urgent agenda we could pursue. This led to the creation of the Outdoor Behavioral Healthcare Research Cooperative (OBHRC) in 1999, with Dr. Keith Russell as director and primary researcher for the first decade. The long-term partnership between the OBH Council and Dr. Russell has resulted in a large body of ground-breaking research on OBH, including outcomes, sustainability of outcomes, beneficial therapeutic factors, and risk incidents.

In 2010, Dr. Michael Gass, University of New Hampshire, was appointed Director of the OBH Research Cooperative. As an academician, Dr. Gass was able to synergize the interest and needs of the OBHC, his academic position and his long-term vision to expand research in the field of Outdoor Behavioral healthcare, with many researchers collaborating on projects and contributing to the growing body of published findings in the field. In 2015, OBHC made the decision to partner with the University of New Hampshire to establish the Outdoor Behavioral Healthcare Center, with Michael Gass as the director and Anita Tucker as associate director. The OBHRC serves "to administer and deliver an active, comprehensive research program on outdoor behavioral healthcare programs operating in North America."

In 2012, OBHC assumed ownership of the annual Wilderness Therapy Symposium, which brings together a broad range of practitioners of wilderness therapy to learn from each other, build a sense of community, and celebrate the field and to disseminate the most recent and significant findings. The symposium continues to expand each year, with its revenues going to support the OBH Center and move forward other initiatives.

In order to promote best practices and establish high standards for membership in OBHC, the council worked with the Association for Experiential Education (AEE) to develop a set of accreditation standards specific to outdoor behavioral healthcare. In 2014, after the standards were developed and approved, the membership agreed to make accreditation with the OBH standards a requirement for all OBHC membership.

Currently at 23 member programs, the OBH Council continues to add new members who embrace its mission. From its humble and uncertain beginning, the Outdoor Behavioral Healthcare Council has fulfilled its vision to create a community of leading programs working together to advance the field through best practices, effective treatment and evidence-based research.

Chapter 10

1996: A History of Summit Achievement
Will White

http://www.summitachievement.com

THE SUMMIT STORY BEGINS WITH AN INTERVIEW with Chris Mays, Adam Tsapis, and Will White filmed on September 12, 2012. The interview started with "tell us the beginnings of Summit Achievement."

Part I

Chris Mays: In 1980, I started working with Outward Bound (OB) on Hurricane Island in Maine. I held a number of positions in the organization and met my wife, Candide Kane, there. At OB we worked with all sorts of populations, including Vietnam Veterans, older people, and teens. But both Candide and I loved working with adolescents with mental health issues. One of the frustrations for us, at the time, was that OB did not have mental health clinicians working with the kids, no family work, and there was no follow up. We still loved it, because we saw the transformative power of the wilderness when angry or disengaged kids completed an OB course and left being positive and open to change for themselves.

In 1987, Candide and I were hired on by OceanQuest; I was employed as a ship's captain. Basically, we were running residential treatment programs on Tall Ships without clinicians on board. I hired Adam Tsapis at that time to be my first mate.

Adam Tsapis: I was drawn to working at OceanQuest because I was a sailor and I had a kinship with some of the students I was working with. Now they were inner city, habitual criminal offenders from Philadelphia, and I was a guy who was kicked out of a boarding school as a kid, but there was a kindred spirit there. I was hired on by Chris as one of the mates. He was a real mentor of mine and inspired me to understand the power of being out in nature and at sea. The importance of the structure and routine was for the students to make change.

Over the years, Chris, Candide, and I talked about starting a program of our own. The kids at OceanQuest were really tough kids and I thought maybe we could work with kids, more like me when I was young, that were making lousy choices, being thrown out of their school, but fundamentally not so self destructive like the kids from OceanQuest. We eventually left OceanQuest and headed up to New England.

Chris Mays: We had a house in New Hampshire and found a great property right over the border in Maine. We started putting together a team of people and we kept hearing about this skilled clinician who worked at a local boarding school. His name was Will White. We got together with him and convinced him to help us start Summit.

Will White: I had been working at a boarding school in New Hampshire when they approached me. Previous to working at the school, I had taken a year off from being a psychotherapist to climb and study Buddhism in different parts of Asia, as I had become disenchanted with traditional outpatient adolescent psychotherapy. When I was at this boarding school, I was excited as I knew I could see the students in all sorts of situations – in dorms, meals, classes. The economy was really bad and school was struggling, so they pretty much enrolled any student whose family could pay full tuition at the school. Needless to say, there was plenty of work for me to help these students get through school without being asked to leave. This was in the early 1990s and there were very few therapeutic schools in the country.

At any boarding school, you have at least two jobs – I ran the outdoor program and was a counselor at the school. So I worked with all these boarding school kids who had previously been at the existing wilderness programs: SUWS, Anasazi, and Aspen Achievement Academy. These kids did great in the outdoor programs that I ran, but at every faculty meeting, the teachers would complain about many of the kids from the wilderness programs saying, "These kids are not ready for the classroom."

So when Chris, Candide, and Adam approached me I said, "This is great, but we have to have an academic component to keep the kids' mindset as students and we have to be licensed as a residential treatment program." There had been a great deal of negative press at the time about wilderness programs. As a clinical social worker trained in family systems, I also felt strongly that parents should interact with their child weekly over the phone or in person with a clinician facilitating.

Adam Tsapis: We ended up calling it Summit Achievement as we were inspired by the mountains that we looked at every day.

Part II

Starting a wilderness program is about building a community of unique individuals around a mission to help young people via the wilderness. People who are referred to as wilderness program "founders" are usually those who have co-signed loans to take on the huge risk of getting a non-traditional business started. Under that definition, Chris Mays, Candide Kane, Adam Tsapis, Will White and Andy Richardson (who trusted us when no bank would) are the founders of Summit. Yet, so many people over its 20 years have helped start, cultivate, and grow Summit to be the excellent program that it is today, there is just not enough space in this chapter to thank them all. To openly express my gratitude, I want to thank everyone who has ever been involved in Summit Achievement for making it the program that it is today. I want to send an invitation to anyone, former student, staff, or family, to our yearly reunion held in October (see Summit Achievement's website for details).

But what is Summit Achievement? Summit Achievement is unique in the field for its integration of the best of evidence-based treatment provided by mental health professionals, accredited academic curriculum, and wilderness therapy. Summit stands out in the modern era of wilderness therapy as it is a "hybrid" program utilizing a campus. Students venture into the field every Thursday and return to the Summit Campus every

Sunday and attend school, sometimes the most challenging part of the week, from Monday to Wednesday.

Summit's campus has a main lodge with administrative offices, a clinician's office, a dining hall, meeting rooms, and logistical areas. There are four cabins that each house up to eight students and two staff and a large academic building that includes five classrooms, plus offices for a physician and nurse, three clinicians, and our academic director. Students attend school Monday, Tuesday, and Wednesday, as well as participate in individual, group, and family psychotherapy. (The family psychotherapy is provided in-person, by phone and via video conferencing.)

Our model of wilderness therapy can be traced directly to Outward Bound's mountaineering-style of expeditions. High-quality gear, team work, and healthy food all are part of our expedition model and have been since day one.

Summit was the first in the field in many ways. Summit was the first program to be licensed by the State of Maine as an adolescent residential treatment center providing mental health and substance abuse treatment and integrating an outdoor component to the program. Summit included family participation in the program, since its inception, which is evidenced by students having weekly family contact – not through letters, but over the phone or through video conferencing throughout their stay in the program. As a regular component of our families' treatment plans, parents come visit their child and take them for an overnight visit into nearby North Conway, New Hampshire and end the visit with a family therapy session on campus.

Summit was also one of the first programs to expand into step-down transitional services, with Summit Semester starting in 2007 (renamed Summit Traverse in 2012). This program was designed to help students transition from wilderness programs to more traditional environments in 2-6 months, such as with an extended academic week, Monday to Friday.

Summit is one of the longest-standing contributors to research in the field of Outdoor Behavioral Healthcare, having contributed our student-based data into a de-identified pool of data, for research by the Outdoor Behavioral Healthcare Council Research Cooperative. Studies by OBHRC and Summit's independent research are available for review on-line (http://www.summitachievement.com/menu/youth-outcome-study). Summit is also one of the few wilderness programs fully accredited by the Association for Experiential Education/Outdoor Behavioral Healthcare Council.

Epilogue

While I am the last of the original founders still at Summit, the program has grown and developed over the past 20 years. It has grown into something I couldn't imagine so many years ago when working in boarding schools. And now, Summit has been achieved and is a place and a culture I have such great pride in. While Chris, Adam, and Candide (see Acknowledgments section) are no longer part of the day-to-day operations, the passion with which we began this program and the vision we helped create, lives on. I can see it through observing a guide staff sitting outside of my window with a student who is tearful after their first parent phone call; or in the spirit of the level movement ceremony I watched today before lunch; or in the camaraderie of a team heading out on expedition. This vision continues to be inspired through the mountains we look at every day.

.

Chapter 11

1997: Soltreks

Lorri Hanna and Doug Sabo

http://soltreks.com

SOLTREKS WAS CO-FOUNDED IN 1997 IN DULUTH, MN. It was easy to create a name for our company. We were clear we wanted to offer an experience that would be the one trek for the soul. After witnessing students as "missed," "lost," or "hidden" within a group setting, we believed we could help students find their spark with a more personal, customized approach toward healing. We chose Duluth, MN as our home and with little resources, we both instructed in the field and provided therapy to students. There were no cell phone or laptop; making a phone call in the woods required the use of a heavy "bag" phone.

When not on trail, we worked part-time or in other wilderness programs to make ends meet. At one point, Lorri was juggling four part-time jobs while establishing an operations and field manual, and Doug was instructing wilderness treks across the country. Although we worked out of our 800 square foot apartment and began with a small business loan of $6800, it was a welcomed challenge to create our vision.

There were a lot of *firsts* with Soltreks. Soltreks was the first wilderness therapy program to offer one-on-one treks at the risk of questions concerning liability and the effectiveness of an individual trek. With diligent risk management, the one-on-one trek proved to be successful. We were also the first wilderness therapy program to offer collegiate internships for Therapeutic Recreation majors, as Lorri is a Nationally Certified Therapeutic Recreation Specialist. Soltreks was the first small wilderness therapy program [the owners were the only two employees] to join OBH Council. Custom family treks, women's treks, young adult treks, parent workshops and sibling work each found their home at Soltreks. Even a group of second year graduate school counseling students spent a week on a custom trek learning counseling tools while discovering their own truths. Soltreks is a program known for its customization.

As Soltreks grew, a summer adventure program sprouted and became one of the primary successful closed-group summer programs in the industry for more than ten years. We believed groups that began and ended together enhance the skills required in a family setting. Quality over quantity preserved the group size, usually no more than six. We also broadened our program area to include New Mexico and Florida. Our growth through the years was also a direct result of our staff, some of the most dedicated and gifted people in the industry. Their feedback consistently polished our manuals and trainings. Staff commitment to our company's mission and best practices has aided Soltreks in maintaining an outstanding safety record. Many (employee) couples met at Soltreks and married!

As founders, we were married to one another and married to our company. Lorri was the Executive Director for 16 years, also supporting admissions, marketing, risk management, staff training, therapist and field instructor. She experienced the outdoors as healing during a personal journey backpacking and hitchhiking cross-country in 1980. She returned to begin a path of learning that included safety/risk management, outdoor leadership and counseling and instructed for programs like Outward Bound or a university's Wilderness Education Association (WEA) course. Lorri has a master's degree in Therapeutic Recreation and is a Licensed Professional Counselor.

Doug's "peak experience" was the spring and summer of 1980 as well, when he and a friend hopped freight trains from California to Minnesota with backpacks in tow, visiting wilderness areas along the way. The connection he found both physically and spiritually to nature inspired his photography and video production work. Doug worked with adjudicated children in a program called Tressler Wilderness School (Pennsylvania, 1990), leading 30-day high impact expedition style wilderness trips. After numerous field days in both the private and public sector and attendance at personal growth retreats, Doug's experience became his education in the therapeutic wilderness field.

Over the years, Soltreks was a board member of several industry professional organizations, presented at national conferences, and mentored new start-up programs. We believed it important to remain educated with the trends in the industry and strive for best practices.

Soltreks has now traveled full circle. Today Doug manages the company solo, offering one-on-one treks to young and older adults. These treks include sea kayaking, canoeing and backpacking. The future will include sailing. Lorri has a new passion and mission. She maintains a spiritual practice of yoga and offers yoga dance and workshops in the community. Lorri continues to offer women's retreats and trekking adventures. She also offers wellness retreats for cancer survivors and their caregivers through art, phototherapy, nature retreats and movement (www.barefootsoulswellness.com, 2014).

Through the years, the integrity of our program, its essence and our commitment never waned. Doug continues to clear the path with the spirit, loyalty and commitment that began in 1997, so others may walk away with a better sense of who they are and who they want to become. As the name suggests, Soltreks truly provides treks for the soul.

Chapter 12

1998:Second Nature: A Mothership

Devan Glissmeyer Ph.D. & Cheryl Kehl LCSW

Co-Founders: Second Nature Wilderness Therapy Program

SecondNaturePrograms.com

In 1997 we believed that a highly clinical model could be integrated into a traditional wilderness program, creating a truly clinical wilderness therapy experience. We knew that primitive living and sophisticated therapy were not mutually exclusive. Primitive living and intense physical/relational challenge just needed to be processed in a way that would shift perspective inward and towards emotional health, and ultimately towards identity and competence. We sat in long meetings that included rich debates over a student's progress being nearly halted if they saw a road or support vehicle. We realized that seeing a road or support truck, let alone a psychologist's visit or psychiatric consult, would not set back progress; it would enhance it. We believed that fresh water could be associated with emotional, cognitive, social and behavioral change. No wilderness programs were delivering fresh water back then. We knew that intense challenge combined with clinical process was commensurate with higher levels of competence. We strove to find the balance between enough challenge and the historic levels of deprivation (that were too often distracting). We pushed past the norm and challenged sacred cows.

Seventeen years ago we believed that we could take the next step in wilderness therapy. When Dan McDougal, Vaughn Heath and we opened the metaphoric doors of our Second Nature Wilderness Therapy Program in Duchesne, Utah (now called Second Nature Uintas) in 1998, we did just that. Having been trained at Aspen Achievement Academy and having learned from the philosophies of Outward Bound, Anasazi, Wilderness Treatment Center and others, we embarked on our own journey.

We were clear that wilderness treatment could be done more effectively, more clinically, and with more customer service. We began writing program philosophies and our own clinical curriculum. We obtained startup loans from family members and started calling Forest Service Rangers to see about obtaining land use permits. Most told us it would be 18 months to get a permit, but Joe Bistrisky, the Ashley National Forest Ranger in Duchesne, Utah, provided us a volunteer work permit in three weeks. He had a nephew who had been in some trouble and Joe understood our hopes. We launched Second Nature on July 1, 1998. We were driving around with a truck and trailer to load up gear, food, and other student needs. We wrote programming and marketing materials while doing every intake and even student transports. We faxed each letter to parents prior to our weekly family therapy calls.

Traditional wilderness treatment at that point was effective, but in our opinion it was not sophisticated and it was not integrated. The wilderness experience was powerful, however, the clinical integration was largely absent, as was the passage of information to referral sources and even to parents. Changes we made included weekly calls to educational consultants to upload information about clinical progress, and more clinical calls to parents, including family therapy components. We hired primarily advanced degree therapists (Ph.D and Ph.D candidates) with expertise in family therapy and adolescent development. We paid them well enough that they stayed on long after they were experts and had developed trusted relationships with referral sources. We provided additional training on the job, often requiring a year of working with another therapist before taking on a full case-load. We required therapists to carry cell phones and be available to families 24/7, knowing that having a child out of the home generates anxiety and other intense emotions.

Our staff were similarly trained, with not only field work instruction and on the job training, but also clinical training, with clinical presentations in staff training, and with the expectation of sitting in on and contributing to therapy sessions with students and their families.

Field instructors became an integral part of the treatment team and helped develop and execute treatment plans.

We began valuing field instructors as critical contributors in the experiential family therapy process. They not only participated at a co-therapy level in individual and group therapy sessions (a departure from the historic top-down model of communication from therapist to field instructor) but also participated in mid program family therapy during parent field visits.

We offered a professional long-term wage in an industry that often relied on paying minimum wage. Field instructors previously often stated that they loved the work but couldn't afford to do it any longer and had to take a higher paying job elsewhere, and would return to the field when they saved enough money. We created a model of customer service that allowed our therapists to be available 24-7 to families and consultants. Previously, the norm was that a therapist was only available one day a week. We changed the model of treatment length from fixed to flexible, helping clients shift from fixations on time to achievement and change. We embraced psychiatric and medication support. We relied on technology and satellite phones to increase safety and begin family therapy from the field. We not only began weekly family therapy phone calls from the field, we asked all parents to come to the field for mid program family therapy. All of these profound changes threatened the 'sacred cows' of prior wilderness therapy culture, when we opened our clinical wilderness doors.

When we reached out to Dr. Brad Reedy to join us, the process of change continued. Along with Dan McDougal and Dr. Ken Newell (and many other brilliant key contributors), we co-founded Second Nature Blue Ridge (the first regional Second Nature program serving the east coast). Then, with Dr. Matt Hoag and Rick Heizer came Second Nature Entrada and with Drs. J and Willow Huffine Second Nature Cascades was created. We were enriched by too many people to list here. The contribution of many was and is felt. Many programs were founded and/or run by Second Nature alumni. Second Nature exists and is better because of the infusion of bright and passionate people. Our industry is better, in part, because of Second Nature's influence and evolution. Our industry is also better because of the evolution of many programs that followed in our footsteps. We are proud of the influence that we've had and grateful for those whose influence we've felt.

Sixteen years ago we set out to create a better experience, for families, employees and referring professionals alike. Last week we had discussions about yet another opportunity to adjust programming to better meet the needs of our students and our families, as we integrated more personalized treatment components into our family therapy model and monthly parent workshops. The evolution continues. We started Second Nature with the goal of creating a better experience and product. We did. From the roots of our origins we continue to grow in health and maturity while branching out to broaden our perspective and experience, from pioneering the flexible length of stay and creating a clinically sophisticated driven model of wilderness therapy to relying on technology and in-field family therapy to integrate family identity work. We are proud of the changes that we induced in our industry. We are proud of our program and our influence. We have succumbed to arrogance at times and been humbled at other times. We have learned life changing lessons from mentors, professional and peers along the way.

Many wonderful and brilliant people have crossed paths with Second Nature. There are few programs that don't have key individuals that worked with us at some point. We are grateful for what we learned and continue to learn. With much respect to those who paved the way ahead of us and for those since who have improved upon our improvements, we continue to evolve and to be grateful for Second Nature and all those who have touched our lives for the positive. We are grateful for the opportunity to "bring families (emotionally) home."©

Chapter 13

1999: History of the Outdoor Behavioral Healthcare Research Cooperative (OBHRC)

Dr. Mike Gass, Dr. Anita Tucker, and Maggie Karoff

http://www.obhcenter.org

O BHRC INITIALLY EVOLVED IN 1999 OUT OF THE efforts of Keith Russell, then a graduate student at the University of Idaho. Keith was interested in coming up with a way to effectively study wilderness therapy participant outcomes as well as risk management patterns in wilderness therapy programs. At the time, the field's reputation was struggling in the media maelstrom that followed a handful of accidents at a few wilderness programs and gravely tarnished the field of wilderness therapy (see Jon Krakauer's *Outside Magazine* article in 1995 October issue titled "Loving Them to Death"). Keith approached a group of individuals involved in the nascent Outdoor Behavioral Health Council to see if he could collect research from the programs. Understanding the importance of research, the OBH Council sponsored the creation of the Outdoor Behavioral Healthcare Research Cooperative (OBHRC). A key visionary for the Cooperative at this time was Dr. Rob Cooley, Executive Director of the Catherine Freer wilderness program. OBHRC was initially created to help Keith research OBH programs in an effort to build a stronger objective empirical base. OBHC programs sent their outcomes data to Keith who analyzed the data. For the first time programs were able to empirically show objective results. Research efforts turned to also focus on risk management data, and Russell provided unprecedented analyses that gave programs a clearer understanding of how and when accidents happened, and steps to become increasingly effective at managing risk in the field.

The evolution of OBHRC and the OBH Center

After nearly a decade at the helm, now Dr. Russell decided in 2009 that his interests were taking him in other directions, and a search began for someone to take over the OBHRC. For many of the same reasons the OBH Council developed a research program, the National Association of Therapeutic Schools and Programs (NATSAP) had already started a research database and network in 2007 under the guidance of Michael Gass, a professor at the University of New Hampshire in the College of Health and Human Services. Dr. Gass saw numerous opportunities in combining the two projects together and jumped at the chance to expand the efforts of both organizations. To this day, the NATSAP Research Database and Network is one of the largest active research databases in the field of behavioral health and substance abuse.

To expand the delivery and quality of research, Dr. Gass needed to attract prolific and qualified researchers that possessed direct knowledge of the field of outdoor behavioral healthcare. The short list that emerged held the very best of current researchers at universities across the country who fit the qualifications of being an OBHRC Research Scientist: (1) a proven researcher holding a tenure-track faculty position at a university, (2) a Ph.D level researcher with an active research agenda, (3) a professional who possessed current clinical licensure in marriage and family therapy, clinical psychology, or social work, and (4) a minimum of two years of "mud on their boots" from direct work experience in outdoor behavioral healthcare. A short list of six other colleagues was created and Dr. Gass called each of researchers to see if they would join him on an exciting journey. From the beginning of making his calls, it took all of 25 minutes to get all of them onboard. These initial conversations with research scientists were straightforward and very exciting. He simply asked, "Do you want to be a part of this?" Everyone seemed to clearly see the enriching value of the opportunity and realized this responsibility would expand their capabilities and their impact.

Possessing clinical expertise, research training, and direct work experience in the field provided this team of researchers a unique ability to ask research questions that had strong potential to improve best practices. This background also enables the researchers to seek out the answers in ways that can meaningfully translate into practice. Between the unique qualifications of researchers and the numerous collaborations between

OBH programs and OBHRC researchers, OBHRC came to embody the reflective researcher-practitioner / practitioner-researcher framework in a powerful way.

The OBHRC research scientists chosen were Dr. Anita Tucker, Associate Professor of Social Work at the University of New Hampshire; Dr. Christine Norton, Associate Professor of Social Work at Texas State University at San Marcos; Dr. Keith Russell, Professor of Recreation at Western Washington University; Dr. Lee Gillis, Professor of Psychology at Georgia College; Dr. Ellen Behrens, Assistant Professor of Mental Health Counseling at Westminster University; Dr. Joanna Bettman Schaefer, Associate Professor and Director of the Masters of Social Work program at the University of Utah; and Dr. Michael Gass, Professor of Outdoor Education at the University of New Hampshire. These individual scientists conduct critically important experiments and also collaborate with the OBHRC research affiliates, researchers who meet most but not all of the research scientist qualifications. Their group efforts have played a critical role in advancing the research efforts on a variety of projects. These individuals are Steve Javorski, Dr. Neal Christianson, Katie Massey, Matt Hoag, and Steve DeMille.

Building upon the success of OBHRC, the OBH Council in conjunction with Dr. Gass and Dr. Tucker at the University of New Hampshire came together to make this partnership more formalized with the creation in June 2015 of the Center for Outdoor Behavioral Healthcare at the University of New Hampshire (www.obhcenter.org). This research center aims to build upon the strong base of OBHRC while also expanding the scope and impact of the OBH within the mental health and substance abuse fields. The OBH Center is working to coordinate and streamline the research efforts of the Research Scientists and affiliated researchers, provide additional opportunities for external funding and collaborations among researchers, exponentially build upon the empirical base of OBH, as well as promote best practices and training in the field. The establishment of the OBH Center is an important step in the validation of the field of Outdoor Behavioral Healthcare.

What questions to ask?

The relationships and partnership built out of the OBHRC and now through the OBH Center allow researchers as well as OBH programs to come together to seek answers to the most critical of questions. Key to their success has been to avoid thinking from a "scarcity point of view" and instead to ask, "What do you want to know?" "If you had all the resources you needed, what questions would you ask?" This often has fueled new research topics as well as critical evaluations of field practices such as using transport services to get youth to programs, as well as the physical impact of OBH programs on youth.

In addition, the questions being asked and researched by OBH Center Research Scientists and affiliated researchers seek to scientifically and objectively take on the questions of justifiably concerned parents. As a parent seeking out treatment for their child, four common questions often emerge:

1. Does it work? Is treatment effective? (Outcome-based research)

2. Is it safe? (Risk management)

3. Is it worth paying for? (Cost effectiveness)

4. How can you tell the good programs from the bad ones? (Program Accreditation)

Note the four answers can be found in the parenthetical listing following these questions. Each of these "answers" serves as one of the four major research foundations of the OBH Center: (1) Outcomes data, (2) Risk management, (3) Cost effectiveness, and (4) Accreditation. These four divisions have become the four legs of the OBH research platform and have provided a general roadmap as OBH Center researchers seek to empirically understand the work of OBH programs.

1. Outcome-based research

While the much of the research produced by the OBHRC and now the OBH Center emanates from the NATSAP database or related projects, it would be misleading to not represent the wide-ranging yet applicable investigations undertaken by the Research Scientists and affiliated researchers. In 2015 alone, over 11 refereed journal articles were published, over 20 research presentations were given both nationally and internationally, and other venues of research reporting in the mainstream press were published. (See appendix or Visit http://www.obhcenter. org/#!bibliography/c106t for a full bibliography of research and resources on OBH).

Generally speaking, most of the data on OBH programs demonstrates that clients experiencing severe problems who enter OBH programs encounter significantly beneficial gains from participation and that these gains are maintained for more than one year after course completion (see Figure 1 below for a representation of OBH data from the NATSAP database, 2015). Recent developments have included major increases in the composite data pool for discharge data six months and one year post-discharge and a new research control group being developed through Redcliff Ascent and Pine River in Canada for upcoming studies.

FIGURE 1.

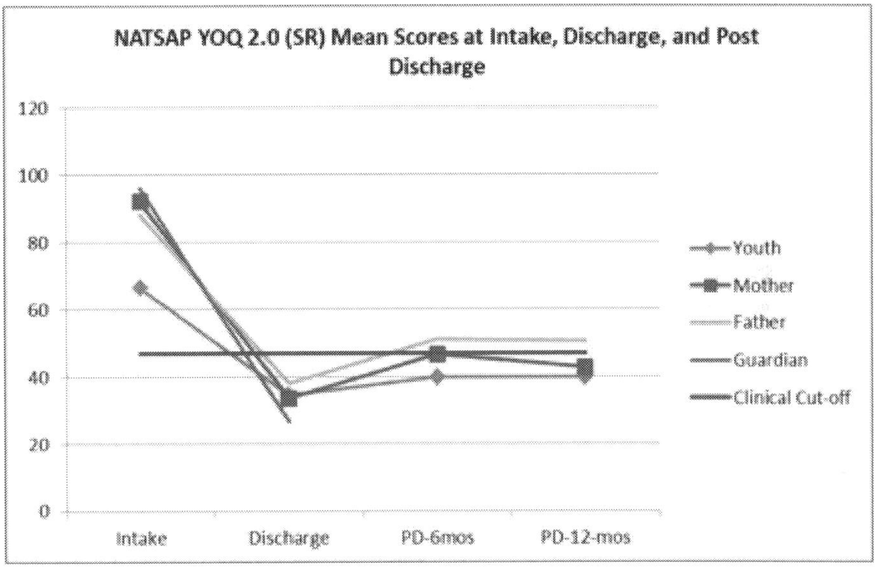

NATSAP YOQ 2.0 (SR) Mean Scores at Intake, Discharge, and Post Discharge

2. Risk Management

Probably no OBH data set is as comprehensive as the risk management data. At the end of December 2014 there were over 20,000 clients in the risk management data set. Besides its size, much of the value of this data is due to the 16+ years of dedicated collection, analyses, and reporting of the OBH Council programs when submitting their data in an accurate, comprehensive, and timely manner. Programs belonging to OBHC have demonstrated that their participants were about two times less likely to visit an emergency room for an injury, than the average American adolescent while in their home community. Figure 2 below illustrates the comparison of OBHC injury rates to those of other common activities.

FIGURE 2.

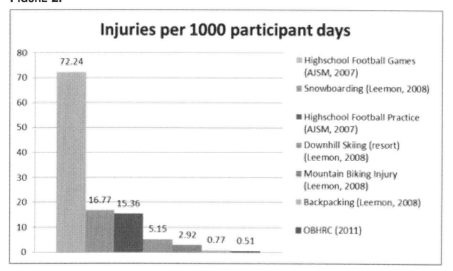

One example comparison is that injuries during high-school football games are over 328 times more common than injuries experienced in OBHC programs. Note that professionals should be careful not to overgeneralize these figures to all wilderness therapy or outdoor behavioral healthcare programs, as this data only represents those reporting program members of the OBH Council.

3. Cost Effectiveness/insurance reimbursement

Assessing the cost effectiveness of OBH often includes a range of questions, including "Is it worth the price?" to "How will it be paid for?" The cost of OBH programs has taken a growing focus of several cost-effectiveness research projects. Over the years, OBHRC and now the OBH Center has supported the work of individuals in the field working to increase reimbursement for OBH programs for families through providing an empirical evidence base for the effectiveness of OBH programs. In 2008, the Mental Health Parity Act paved the way to advocate with increased vigor for insurance companies to pay for wilderness therapy. Since this time, over $1.2 million have been received by families to partially or totally cover the costs of OBH programming. The hope is that in the future, OBH becomes a nationally recognized and reimbursed treatment option for youth and young adults.

4. Program accreditation

Recently, the OBH Council and the Association of Experiential Education (AEE) embarked upon a thorough examination of OBH standards to better reflect the field's current practices. This resulted in a voluntary credentialing program for OBH providers, where programs are scrutinized by a team of experts in the field. Accredited OBH programs have demonstrated they operate at or above industry-leading standards of ethical care, treatment evaluation, and risk-management practices. The AEE OBH accreditation process began in the Fall of 2014, and has become a requirement of membership in OBHC. The first accreditation site visits – Open Sky, Anasazi, and Summit Achievement – were powerful experiences. Watching programs open their doors and let in colleagues who are their competitors to critique them is a true testament to the spirit of collaboration, openness, and transparency in the partnership between OBHC programs and the OBH Center.

The future of OBH Center

The true value of OBH research lies in its utility and value in shaping the field. When done right, research can serve as a "moral compass." Research has the capacity to give a true direction, not pulled by the diverting forces of politics or financial constraints, but rather guided by the true perspective of the answers to the questions we ask. While the day-to-day experience of OBH Center researchers often involves calculating numbers, delving through documents, responding to phone calls and generating statistical models, the bigger picture of this work is when parents call us in the office, as they often do, we are able to objectively say, "this will help your child get better, and here is how we know." We work with incredible people in this field, amazing individuals who are passionate about achieving their dreams, about always improving practices and continually raising the bar, about helping kids and families heal. The members of OBHC trust the work of the OBH Center and its researchers; and it is a privilege to work with these individuals, to be part of this community, and to do research that has such a direct impact on the lives of families and youth.

Chapter 14

2000: SUWS of the Carolinas

Rebecca Vines

http://suwscarolinas.com

Suws of the Carolinas is nestled in a remote part of Old Fort, North Carolina, surrounded by the Blue Ridge Mountains. The drive to SUWS requires going on long, windy back roads. Cars normally have to stop for turkeys crossing the roads. There is a bridge above a rushing creek that all staff and visitors have to walk over in order to get to the SUWS base camp. To the left there is a pond filled with frogs, fish, and sometimes turtles and water snakes. To the right there is a field lined with rustic cabins with a large oak tree in the middle. It is the perfect setting for a wilderness program.

In the spring of 2000 when Jim Gleaser, Reid Treadaway, Bob Hanna, Jack Kline, and Todd Walker walked over the bridge to SUWS of the Carolinas, things looked very different. There were no cabins lining the field. It was not uncommon to see a staff member or a dog swimming in the pond. Students were just starting to arrive in North Carolina for treatment in the wilderness.

SUWS of the Carolinas was founded in the year 2000 by Aspen Education Group. SUWS of Idaho had been open since 1981 and was thriving. At the time, there were a number of Wilderness Therapy companies located on the West coast. Many students were flying all the way from New York and Boston to attend SUWS Idaho. The idea to open a program on the East Coast started forming. Wouldn't it be so much easier for parents in New England to fly or drive their children to a closer program in the same time zone?

Jim Glaeser started working for SUWS Idaho in 1994 as a Field Instructor. He was drawn to the program by his love for the outdoors as well as working with teenagers. After working as a Field Instructor, he worked as a Field Supervisor and then was the Assistant Director for several months. During his time as the Assistant Director, Jim was asked to help start up SUWS of the Carolinas as the Executive Director. Before long he was in Old Fort, North Carolina interviewing staff to work for him.

Reid Treadaway was working in admissions for the CEDU programs in Idaho when he heard about the opening of SUWS of the Carolinas. Being from South Carolina, the idea of moving back East and having the opportunity to continue to work with teenagers was appealing to him. His degree in Forest Management is how he initially became involved in working with kids. He loved teaching them about nature. Reid called SUWS of the Carolinas and asked if they needed someone to work in their admissions department. At that point, the admissions department was in Gooding, Idaho so it was perfect timing on Reid's part. He moved to North Carolina and set up the first admission office in Old Fort.

Bob Hanna has always had a love for nature and outdoors. He was introduced to Wilderness Therapy when he was in graduate school and began his career with Aspen Achievement Academy in 1992. In 2000, Bob was in working in Salt Lake City but he and his wife were interested in moving to Asheville, North Carolina and he was actively searching for a job there. He found the clinical director position for SUWS on the internet. With the combination of Wilderness Therapy and Asheville, Bob thought it was meant to be.

Jack Kline started his career in Wilderness Therapy in Miami working with high risk teenagers at an adventure based counseling program. He had worked with the Miami police department gang unit to get kids back on the right track. The program incorporated wilderness elements such as a high ropes course. Jack was living in Asheville, working in therapeutic foster care when he saw an ad in the paper for a therapist position at SUWS. He spoke to Jim and started as one of the first therapists at SUWS.

Todd Walker became interested in Wilderness Therapy after taking a year long intensive course in Outdoor Leadership. He started his career in Wilderness Therapy in 1995 and in 2000, he was field instructing at SUWS of Idaho. That summer, Todd received a call from Jim who asked if he and his wife were interested in moving to Asheville to work at SUWS of the Carolinas.

SUWS of the Carolinas officially enrolled the first student in May, 2000. Jim, Bob, and Jack, along with a few other staff were there to see the first group form. Todd arrived to work as the Field Director in June. At that time there were 6 adolescent students enrolled. They were all in the same co-ed group. Reid started in September of 2000. He remembers the day that he walked over the bridge to SUWS and was shown to his office. He opened the door and saw a completely empty office. "There was no desk and no chairs. There wasn't a computer. It was just an empty office." That's how new the program was.

That summer, SUWS of the Carolinas mirrored SUWS of Idaho. Reid spent some time training at the admissions office and in the field in Idaho. Jim and Todd had both spent years working at SUWS Idaho. Staff taught students wilderness and survival skills. The curriculum was similar to the Idaho program, but focused more on the unique terrain of North Carolina's course areas. SUWS of the Carolinas grew quickly and changed quickly.

In the beginning all of the students started and finished the program at the same time. Soon this changed to rolling admissions. This was a completely different model that staff had to adapt to. Students also started staying in the program longer. As with most start-ups the original team transitioned out and a new set of directors came on board through the years. In the spring of 2003, Graham Shannonhouse came over from SUWS Idaho and became the Executive Director. Under her leadership, SUWS continued to grow and develop over the years, adding a youth program in 2004 with Leah Madamba as the Program Director, and then a parent centered Family Program with Dr. Brooke Judkins. SUWS of the Carolinas began to thrive as a leader in creative and specialized program and quickly began to grow into one the largest wilderness therapy programs in the country.

Shawn Farrell originally came to SUWS of the Carolinas in 2003, and returned as the Executive Director in 2008 and has continued this drive to create treatment specific niche programs, with SUWS now offering four different programs and the family program. These unique programs are available so that our students can get the specific clinical treatment that they need. Our SUWS program consists of adolescent male and females, ages 13-17, grouped by gender. The Seasons program is geared towards our younger students ages 10-13. The Approach program works students ages 13-17 living with autism spectrum disorders and struggling with social issues. The Phoenix program is our recovery program working with 13-17 year old students struggling with substance abuse. Field Instructors working in these groups get specific training for the population they are working with. Program Managers and Therapists teach these staff specialized skills and tools so they can provide excellent, relevant care.

Though originally SUWS mirrored the Idaho "nomadic" model, it now operates using a base camp model. There are cabins that students rotate through for sleeping and they are always available during inclement weather. The first sets of cabins were added in 2003 due to a change in North Carolina licensure of the program, and then more were added as the demand for the program grew. A second base camp was built for the Phoenix program in 2006 & 2007 to house students between their field expeditions; Phoenix students make use of these base camp days practicing yoga and therapeutic drumming, attending NA meetings, working on academics, and utilizing neurofeedback.

Over the past decade SUWS has strived for excellence and continues to implement change to make the program more successful. SUWS is now academically accredited by AdvancED as a school and students receive academic credits upon graduation. SUWS is accredited by CARF and is licensed by the NC division of Health Service regulation. Over the years Canine Therapy and Equine Assisted Therapy became integrated into the programs, offering further therapeutic access and growth for our students.

Although SUWS of the Carolinas has changed a lot over the years, many things are still the same. The most important thing that has not changed is our mission, which is summed up in our mission statement that the community of SUWS created together in 2010. "Through the wilderness, we empower families to discover their strengths by creating a safe and consistent environment to restore hope and foster growth."

Chapter 15

2001: Outback Therapeutic Expeditions

Rick Meeves Ph.D.

https://www.outbacktreatment.com

OUTBACK THERAPEUTIC EXPEDITIONS, ORIGINALLY known as Walkabout Therapeutic Expeditions, was founded by myself (Rick Meeves) and Tim Thayne, with the gifted and capable assistance of Shayne Gallagher and Michael Bednarz.

Outback started as a small, therapeutic wilderness program in May 2001. It was founded on the basis of clinical excellence and sophistication along with a strength-based, relationship-driven, and strong family model.

My professional background included a Masters in Marriage and Family Therapy from the University of Nebraska and my doctorate from Brigham Young University. After completing my doctoral internship, I was recruited by Dr. Brad Reedy, who at the time worked at Aspen Achievement Academy. It was there that I cut my first teeth as a wilderness therapist and trained under the direction of Dr. Paul Goddard. After two years at Aspen Achievement Academy, I accepted a job as Clinical Director at Aspen Ranch. After serving several months, it became necessary for me to leave Aspen Ranch and become a stay-at-home dad while finishing my doctoral dissertation. Six months later I accepted an offer to work at Second Nature, in Duchesne, Utah, and remained employed there for two years. In 2001, I convinced a few amazing people to join my cause and started Walkabout Therapeutic Expeditions.

Dr Tim Thayne and I knew each other from our undergraduate days and remained in contact throughout our graduate studies in MFT. Tim earned his masters in MFT from BYU and his Ph.D from Virginia Tech. He was working in his family business and running a small consulting company when I approached him to consider helping start Walkabout/ Outback. He agreed and helped fund our little start up and after 18 months joined full-time, taking a caseload and helping with marketing and the business office.

Shayne Gallagher also helped start Outback. His primary duties included field directing and designing the curriculum, with its unique token system, and fabulous staffing model, as well as teaching the parent seminar. Shayne's background included many years in this field, including work at Anasazi, Second Nature, and a wilderness/residential start up in Logan, Utah.

Mike Bednarz also was instrumental in helping Walkabout/Outback get off the ground. His masters degree and background in education and logistics, along with time as a field staff and academics director at Second Nature-Duchesne, were an excellent coupling to Shayne's experience in helping with policies and procedures, staff manuals, logistics, field staff training, licensing, and academics.

Inspiration

The inspiration and origins of Walkabout/Outback were two-fold. In an interview that was posted on our website, I explained that "we combined the best of modern clinical practices and the best of wilderness programming for teens to create a very viable, relationship-driven and clinically-based model that was less behavioral than other wilderness models and more focused on internal change and internal locus-of-control."

Another unique feature was the location in the west desert of Utah, which allowed therapists to do their fieldwork while returning to their homes and families at night. This was a difference from other wilderness programs in Utah that required therapists to be out of town for 3 to 4 days a week to complete field work.

Finally, our family programming was exceptional and offered an alternative to the traditional graduation ceremonies that families would attend. Outback systematically requested families to attend a mid-stay parent visit and parent seminar which facilitated a significant amount of face-to-face family therapy and reality testing for both the parents and the teen prior to the euphoria that often accompanies the end-of-stay graduation ceremonies at most wilderness programs. This mid-stay visit helped deemphasize the sense of students "completing" treatment and placed higher emphasis on the notion of continuing treatment. The intent was to reduce the transitional stresses and regression that can frequently occur when teens transition to therapeutic boarding schools or residential treatment centers. Furthermore, it helped increase the amount of reality testing necessary for those teens transitioning to home, by exposing them to the breakdowns in communication that can occur during any family therapy session.

Outback utilized a unique model that engaged the teens in making multiple primitive objects such as an external frame backpack, Bow-drill fireset, moccasins, leather "possibles bag" to carry their books and letters, pottery, small medicine or keeper pouch necklace, a Native American flute, Australian-based Didgeridoo, and a dozen other items. The beauty of this model emphasized the notion of "inviting inquiry" where students would engage in the therapeutic process rather than simply resist rules or require pursuit by the staff and therapists. Outback also utilized an elaborate token system (not like a token economy) with designs on sixteen different wood burned tokens that rewarded students for progress in their specific areas. This strength-based system was devised as an alternative to the traditional level systems that often allow teens to jump through hoops and manipulate staff and programs. These programmatic elements constituted the reasons for starting Outback, namely that we felt there was room for an alternative to the more behavioral, level-system type therapeutic wilderness programs.

What is Going on Today

In order to explain what is going on today at Outback, it is necessary to retrace a few steps.

In 2004, Walkabout Therapeutic Expeditions was approached and acquired by the Aspen Education Group. Shortly after the acquisition, Walkabout changed its name to Outback Therapeutic Expeditions. It continued to grow through 2007 when the Aspen Education Group was acquired by the CRC Health Group. During the recession in 2008, Outback experienced a reduction in size like most wilderness programs, but continued to survive up until 2013 when it began to experience turnover in key therapists and difficulty in rebuilding under CRC's ownership. In August 2014, after struggling to recover, CRC inquired about my interest in purchasing Outback. Instead of allowing Outback to be closed, I purchased Outback in September 2014. Shortly thereafter, I entered a partnership with the Aspiro group, attained the next generation of leadership at Outback, and it continues to regain momentum, providing great service to families and teens and referral sources, consistent with its historically strong clinical and relationship focus. Outback has remained strong to its roots but also plans to roll out some program enhancements in 2015.

Chapter 16

2003: Wilderness Therapy Symposium

Rob Meltzer

https://obhcouncil.com/symposium

IT WAS LATE SEPTEMBER, 2003 AND IT WAS A BEAUTIFUL evening in Boulder, Colorado. The energy was electric. There was a playful spirit in the air and people were wondering what this new event was all about. So was I. I had no idea what was about to emerge.

On that first evening of the Wilderness Therapy Symposium, about 160 people packed into the Performing Art Center on the Main Campus at Naropa University in Boulder, CO. I had only one agenda. I wanted to open a 'space' where we could share our love for working with people in the outdoors. To bring the spirit of nature into the room, we sat in silence for a moment, took a bow of intention, and then Naropa students shared songs and poetry. When I stepped up on the stage, people seemed calm yet eager. I implored the audience to leave their marketing agenda at the door, to open their minds and hearts, to really listen to each other, and to allow themselves to have an experience with nature. I gave the definition of a Symposium: "A meeting for discussion of a topic, especially one in which the participants form an audience and make presentations." The intention for the event was to teach each other what we have learned ourselves from Mother Nature.

People were ready to share and they jumped right in. Deborah Bowman, Deb Piranian, Bill Plotkin, and Gary Ferguson were our featured speakers. Their words resonated and set a vibe that is still imprinted on the event today. When Gary spoke, I remember feeling as though Mother Nature herself had entered the room and was bestowing her gifts on us.

Deb Piranian captured the spirit of the event best when she said that "we are here to cross pollinate the worlds." Like bees sharing bits of pollen, we shared our wisdom and our passion with each other. We wove together an immensely diverse audience and somehow the differences ended up being the strength of the event.

Perhaps the most radical idea was to run a conference that would take over 150 people to nearby wilderness for daylong workshops. We had no budget to hire transportation, so it became an enormous carpool. It was insane, but we pulled it off!

By the time the first Symposium was complete, people felt that something special had just happened. People had come together cooperatively to co-create a learning environment. We shared intimately, openly, and deeply. From then on, the spirit of collaboration was infused into the Symposium and still exists today.

Now, in 2015, the WTS is a national conference that attracts close to 500 people. "It consists of interactive presentations, speakers and outdoor experiential workshops and brings a diverse cross-section of clinicians, field instructors, rites of passage guides, educational consultants, professors, research specialists, students and residential program staff under one roof to share theories, insights and best practices in an open spirit. The symposium is a place to explore, inform, and educate ourselves on a diverse range of topics all centering on the healing power of wilderness." (from the WTS website).

The original idea for the Wilderness Therapy Symposium came to me, in 2002, during a committee meeting at Naropa University. At the time, I was the Director of the Transpersonal Counseling Program (TCP) and we had just launched the new Master's Program in Wilderness Therapy and an online Ecopsychology degree program. I wanted to present these new programs to the world. So, I decided to create an interactive and informative event where people could have a therapeutic experience in nature. Rather than just talk about Wilderness Therapy, we would experience it. I decided to call the event a Symposium and set an intention of sharing and collaboration.

I invited everyone I knew who loved working with people in the outdoors. Because of my background, that was a large and eclectic group. Early in my career, I worked in Adventure Education programs such as the Boojum Institute, Four Corners School, and Deer Hill Expeditions.

In the mid 90's, I obtained a Master's Degree in Counseling Psychology with a concentration in Wilderness Therapy from Prescott College. Right out of grad school, I became the Principal of a special needs charter school, called Community of Learners, that used Outdoor Education as the primary pedagogy. Over the years, I worked in spiritually-based programs such as Animas Valley Institute. I also trained as a Wilderness Therapist with Roger Strachan at the Southwest Association for Gestalt and Expressive Studies and Wilderness Encounter.

In the mid-90's I started teaching a class at Naropa University called The Psychology of Wilderness Experience. In 2000, I launched my Educational Consulting practice and was concurrently hired as the Director of the Transpersonal Counseling Department. Deborah Bowman, Chair of the Transpersonal Counseling department, had a vision for a Master's Program in WT and asked me to help her get it off the ground. The consulting business and program development work at Naropa helped me become intimately familiar with the Wilderness Therapy programs that now populate NATSAP and OBH Council.

This is how it came to be that the original invitation went out to a large and diverse group of adventure-based educators, wilderness therapists, professors, field guides, program owners, administrators, students, rites of passage guides, researchers, and visionaries. They were simply the people I had met along the way and I was inviting them to celebrate our passion for working with people outdoors.

When I hit 'Send' on that first invite, I had no idea what was about to happen. I was blown away by the response. People loved the idea and offered all sorts of assistance. Programs contributed money and committed to send staff. Students volunteered. Friends, colleagues, and family came out of the woodwork to help me.

The Symposium has always had a life of its own. Over the years, the event evolved and grew into a major national conference managed by the Outdoor Behavioral Healthcare Council. The OBH Council is a non-profit organization dedicated to raising the bar in the field of Wilderness Therapy by conducting research and helping programs implement standards and best practices. OBH Council is emerging as the industry's leader and their partnership with the Symposium is synergistic. There are now committees which organize and manage the event and it is inclusive of a much wider group of professionals in the field. It is wonderful to see the investment that so many people put into it each year!

There is one person who has remained a steady, behind-the-scenes force and who is responsible for making the Symposium what it is today. That person is Jim Lavin. As Event Coordinator, he manages all of the logistics and details and makes it all happen with grace and kindness. The Symposium would simply not be what it is without Jim's steady hand holding it all together.

The Symposium is a big metaphorical campfire that people love to gather around. It brings together a diverse crowd and connects them around a common love for Nature. My hope is that it will always be about collaboration and never about marketing.

Chapter 17

2004: Pacific Quest

Suzanne McKinney

http://www.pacificquest.org

THERE IS A SENSE OF PRIDE AND ACCOMPLISHMENT in being able to write the history of our program from the first person perspective. For 10+ years, we have all been answering frequent and similar questions about our origin. Everything from, "How did you get into THIS business," to "Why Hawaii?" to "When will you be going back to the mainland?" A decade later, we are humbled by our journey, and we remain dedicated to bringing innovative, sustainable care to our families.

Mike and Suzanne McKinney and Chris Kaiser opened Pacific Quest (PQ) in January of 2004. Mike is a passionate, visionary man; anyone would agree. With incredible strategic abilities, he is able to create and manage our multi-faceted and developing program. It is his fearless, open-minded approach that has allowed PQ to be progressive and sustainable for 10 years.

Chris Kaiser makes things happen. He is tireless in his efforts to find the best way, the smartest approach to a challenging situation. A kind heart and a passion for the search for meaning drives him and his contributions to PQ. Chris' intent to do the right thing for adolescents and YA's and to help them find their place in the world drives the soul of PQ.

Suzanne is our "outside voice." She blends her program support with her natural relationship skills in order to communicate our unique program philosophy and message. Even amidst our growth, she continues to promote and uphold the sophisticated nature and the purpose of our program.

The three founders met in Idaho at the SUWS program in 1999. Mike and Chris were field instructors in the 21-day, primitive skills, Search and Rescue model program for 2 years. Suzanne was providing aftercare options for students who had completed the SUWS program. Each founder came to Idaho in search of growth and challenge, personally and professionally.

While Suzanne was working closely with parents, referral sources and other therapeutic programs, Mike and Chris spent many hours in the field observing and scrutinizing the model within which they were working with adolescents. It was an early dream to create their own effective, unique and meaningful outdoor therapeutic program.

A crucial influence to PQ was Chris' Rites of Passage (ROP) training with the School of Lost Borders. After his first Vision Fast with SOLB, he knew clearly that he wanted to merge what he was learning with ROP with the population he had been working with for years at SUWS. Wilderness Therapy for Adolescents seemed very fertile ground for ROP work because most programs already incorporated some sort of solo component into the program. There was a general understanding that reflective time alone in nature was a good thing, but he didn't see anyone using it as intentionally or as substantially as SOLB was.

Mike and Chris began to collaborate on independent wilderness therapy "ventures" outside of SUWS. They customized trips with wilderness therapy alumni and individual families that included primitive skills, backpacking and increasingly, Rites of Passage. These trips culminated in a successful group trip to Western Samoa for a month, where they recognized the benefit of a safe physical environment and the importance of culture that Samoa provided.

Upon return, Chris, Mike and Suzanne began the discussion and ultimately took the plunge, starting their own therapeutic, land-based program in Hawaii. They all had ideas about a unique new approach to Wilderness Therapy that incorporated the best of what they had learned along the way and yet were quite distinctive.

Starting out in Hawaii was unique to the wilderness therapy community, and them, and, as they learned, very new to the people and communities in Hawaii. Chris, Mike and Suzanne were certain that it was important to remain open to what this new land and culture had to teach them. This was not a simple case of duplicating a survival model from the Idaho high desert! It was in clearing the land, working with the first few students, learning from the Hawaiian people, and a having a desire for change that they developed the PQ model. Having a heightened awareness of their surroundings, they soon were able to cultivate an impactful and effective program in Hawaii utilizing ROP, agriculture, Hawaiian culture and wellness.

The vision was to create a controlled and safe outdoor environment in which to experience, practice and develop new ideas and skills. They aimed to create an environment where blame and excuses could not get in the way of true internal change. They developed a program that dismissed manufactured and coerced scenarios for natural consequences and true desire for change. The balance between the knowledge they brought with us to Hawaii and being open to Hawaii's gifts allowed them to tap into Hawaii's abundant cultural richness and the unique historical relationship between the people and the land.

They chose a small, rural campus on seven acres and quickly discovered organic farming provided the focus, metaphors and congruency with traditional Hawaiian sustainable agriculture that would provide the foundation for the program. For the students at Pacific Quest, the process of change and growth that they witness in the garden provides an opportunity to look more closely at the change and growth taking root within themselves.

Over the years, they have integrated wellness into the Pacific Quest core program. They realized that physical health, including nutrition, movement and self-care is essential to the sustainable success of the students. Students grow and eat organic, local food, learn healthy eating and sleeping habits, and study the relationship between mind and body. Maintaining this piece of the program has proven to be one of the most innovative and valuable achievements.

Today, Pacific Quest has grown to include three more properties, and a thriving Young Adult program. They are able to serve up to 100 students at a time, 365 days a year, from all over the world. Although the staff and facilities have grown, the founders' intent has not wavered. As owners and operators, they are steadfast in their vision. In the last few years, they have recommitted themselves and the program to the mission:

Pacific Quest cultivates sustainability in our students, in our families, in our communities, and in ourselves.

Chapter 18

2005: True North Wilderness Program
Madhurii Barefoot

http://truenorthwilderness.com

T

RUE NORTH WILDERNESS PROGRAM ENROLLED its first student on a snowy December day, in 2005 in a small, quaint New England village in a bucolic valley tucked alongside the Green Mountains. The valley is where I grew up and my family still lives here. In many ways, the story of True North is an extension of my life and the life and journey of Ty Maves, my husband and co-founder of True North.

Ty and I met in 1999 at SUWS. Ty had attended the University of Montana and completed and undergraduate degree in Psychology. He drove over to SUWS from Bend, Oregon to satisfy his curiosity about wilderness therapy. I had recently graduated from Smith College and had planned to drive to Wyoming to attend a NOLS instructor course. I had participated in a NOLS semester in Patagonia during a gap year and thought I might put my job interviews with Manhattan publishing houses on hold and lead some NOLS courses. A friend suggested that I stop off at SUWS on my way. I decided I could broaden the adventure of driving West and steer my trusty Subaru to Idaho, a place I had never been before.

Far from the potato fields I expected, the Bennett hills of Idaho turned out to be a stunning landscape of deep desert canyons scented with sagebrush and juniper, framed by the Sawtooth mountains, and populated with coyotes, rattlesnakes, and, as it turned out, struggling teenagers from all over the world. Ty and I would spend the next several years leading trips in Idaho and eventually at SUWS of the Carolinas.

We immersed ourselves in the world of wilderness therapy. We soaked up the stories and the experience of mentors like Dennis Thompson who taught us how to make drums with goatskins and how to find wild edibles. More importantly, he and many other inspiring individuals taught us how to truly listen to and connect with our students, how to help them face their pain and confusion while coaxing the very best from them to show them a small kernel of the future that could be theirs if they were willing to accept support and move forward. We lay gazing at the stars in the desert dreaming of what our own program might someday be like.

In 2003 we completed our graduate degrees in Oregon and returned to SUWS in Idaho as therapists. After a few years, I began to feel a longing for the East coast, for fall foliage and apple cider, for small communities tucked into wooded mountain valleys. After evaluating all of our dreams we agreed that we could not imagine walking away from the profound richness and satisfaction of working in this field.

Andy Chapman, close friend and wilderness guide extraordinaire called from Idaho and insisted that we could do it. "I'll come out to help for a couple of months," he said, and within a few weeks he had arrived in Vermont where he stayed for over two years. My childhood friend Kate Weir had earned a business degree and was looking for an opportunity to contribute to a new project. The four of us spent hours around our kitchen table envisioning every aspect of our program. Digging into the well of our collective knowledge we identified our mission statement: to be the cornerstone of positive change for our students and their families.

We defined our ideal clients, articulated admissions criteria and drafted a curriculum rooted in self-reflection and personal development. We agreed that our program should be small so that we could individualize our work, appreciating and responding to the unique needs of each student and their family. We wanted to share with our clients the sense of community and support that we feel is essential to becoming a good citizen in the world and that is one of the many joys of living in our small community in Vermont.

We incorporated our love of outdoor adventure by outfitting our students with high quality gear and clothing, a dramatic departure from the more spare and primitive model we had been trained in. We crafted the metaphor of our model and chose the language that would become our program's vernacular carefully, agonizing over the names of each task and phase. We envisioned a program that would promote maturity and independence, confidence and leadership. We built a program environment that was familiar and accessible to many of our prospective families and one that could wrap our students in the cozy green hills and valleys of Vermont.

The ideas flew, we would take our students skiing, we would sleep in heated shelters in the winter, no more freezing nights wrapped in a plastic bedroll on the snow. We would create phases that were developmental and that would give our students some way to measure and contextualize their progress, we would keep therapist caseloads small, providing a concentrated therapeutic experience. We created a program that married our clinical training with the more experiential and environmentally driven work that had captured our hearts in the Bennett hills of Idaho.

Most of the early concepts generated around our kitchen table have become central to our program and our process. Other ideas have been modified or retired, like the fancy backpacking pillows that our first students complained were really just not necessary. Some additions were carefully wrought and built in organized phases. Others were the result of serendipitous connection-a sequence of ideas organically building and culminating in some new aspect of our program.

Our first client was approaching her 18th birthday and came to True North in part to prepare for her transition to young adulthood. As part of her work, her educational consultant Rob Meltzer and I decided to collaborate and invite her parents to our office for a weekend workshop. It was a profound experience. We had moved far beyond the didactic presentation, a million miles away from a whiteboard filled with generic concepts. It seemed natural to offer this experience to all of our clients. Rob collaborated with us until Caretia Fernandez took over the parent program.

Caretia had first visited True North in the fall of 2006. We connected instantly, and by February of 2007 Caretia had joined our team. She is not only a gifted therapist but also a visionary and she took our original parent workshop model and grew it into a comprehensive integrated parent program. Now we have an entire team of dedicated parent therapists. I cannot imagine True North without our parent program, it is so central to our identity and such a cherished part of the work we do. We have been lucky enough to welcome many extraordinary individuals, like Caretia, who have shaped the program and have contributed their own particular stamp to the culture and community of True North.

Early on, Ty, Andy, Kate and I wore many hats, shopping for oatmeal and sleeping bags and used Suburbans, writing curriculum and changing tires. Mike Balotti joined us a year after Caretia to become our first Admissions Director. Mike quickly became indispensible and has coached hundreds of families through the conversations that begin their journey here, and he has been a key member of our administrative team. Mike is passing the Admissions torch to Courtney Merrill and we know this marks an important new chapter for our program. Courtney is a gifted clinician and brings with her a wealth of experience and insight-we know she will have much to contribute to our program and our field.

Over the years we have accumulated a "brain trust" of assorted professionals. Educators, nutritionists, clinical professionals, foresters, wildlife biologists and more who have helped us to do everything from expanding our field areas to revamping our menu. Some critical improvements have included the acquisition and development of our winter campus, and the addition of our young adult program.

We have watched proudly and reaped the benefits as our staff pursued their personal and professional development. When our program director Ben Loveless completed his master's in Environmental Education last year, we celebrated by handing him the entire student curriculum to edit and update. We have been thrilled to welcome back as therapists multiple folks who began their careers in wilderness therapy here and have come "home" after completing their education and gaining experience in the field. Every one of our field directors and logistics managers have been guides here first, and now they add their rich personal knowledge of our mission and work to every aspect of our daily operation.

We have celebrated so many families and new babies here at True North in the past few years that we invested in True North onesies and learned how to set up 529 college savings plans. We have welcomed many international students and will travel to multiple countries in the coming months to share our work with colleagues from London to Singapore. As it was in the very beginning, swapping stories and ideas around our kitchen table, True North's greatest strength is our community. Our community of gifted and caring staff, our amazing clients and their families, the beautiful Vermont valley that we call home and the citizens of the global community that find their way to the Green Mountains.

Chapter 19

2005: Open Sky Wilderness Therapy: A History

Aaron Fernandes

http://www.openskywilderness.com

"**A**RE YOU STILL IN?" WAS THE QUESTION AARON Fernandes asked, with hope and excitement, of his start up team in August, 2005. When they had accepted his invitation to be part of starting an innovative new wilderness therapy program, the proposal had included a partner with a million dollars of start-up money. Now Aaron was calling to say plans had changed: no more partner, no more investment capital.

Eight months prior, an investor looking for a meaningful yet lucrative investment opportunity had approached Aaron and asked if he wanted to start a wilderness therapy program; the question was intriguing and well timed. After five years of working for corporately owned programs, Aaron had been working on plans to start his own independent wilderness program.

Over those eight months Aaron and the investor developed strategy, explored potential locations, and hosted key employee recruits in the chosen home of Durango, CO. On a sunny weekend in May, 2005 Aaron pitched the vision for how this program would be very different: offer not only excellent clinical programming, but organic foods, naturopathic medicine, psychiatry, yoga, meditation, research, and intensive family services.

As the planned start date drew closer, spreadsheets, numbers, and analysis ensued. It became clear how expensive the multi-disciplinary model would be to operate. Tension followed. "Organic food is great, but let's spend more on food once we establish ourselves," said the investor. "Family programming is needed, but why offer more than our competitors for the same rate?" "I don't see how we can justify the cost of research: it will be ten years before we have meaningful results." And finally, "Let's start with the basics and add more later."

Yet Aaron's vision of a holistic, health and family oriented program was not one he could walk away from easily. He had found Aspen Achievement Academy, the flagship wilderness therapy at the time, in 1999 and worked for several years as a field instructor. He believed in the power of food as medicine, and had seen how powerful the connection between food and health was from gardening with inner city kids in his university town of Providence, Rhode Island. He believed in meditation and mindfulness, practices that had been life changing for him during post college his travels in India. And he believed that family should be more included in the process. After this time Aaron became Field Director at Aspen and then Executive Director for a program in Montana. He tried to implement his ideas for holistic and family programming in these settings but was curbed by the realities of working for a large corporation.

So while the investor's offer of start up money was compelling, so was the reality of signing over 51% of the control. For Aaron it was both agonizing and clear: he'd rather risk the venture altogether than give up influence of his vision and values.

He declined the offer. After months of sharing such excitement and possibility it was a personal loss for them both. Yet there was mutual understanding and the parting was amicable.

Which led to the phone call to ask of his recruits, "Are you still in?" and affirmation when all five replied, enthusiastically, "Yes!"

While the start-up team had passion and years of experience in wilderness therapy as field instructors, therapists, administrators, and directors, they did not have capital. Aaron's modest personal savings was not enough to launch a program. To keep the vision moving forward he had to secure funding.

Aaron sought out a cross section of local, regional, state and federal banks and presented his business plan. The bankers were skeptical. "The client population is risky." "Your holistic model is unproven." "The majority of the loan money you are requesting goes to salaries. We'll need assets if you fail." All ten bankers said no.

Aaron was disappointed, and, perhaps naively, surprised. Yet he stayed on the path, which brought him to a local economic development agency. He made a case: the business would create 25 new jobs out of the gate and with time that number would grow. Not only would it infuse money into the local economy, it would do good. The loan was approved.

While a boon, the loan was far from a million dollars. The pressure was on. The team worked round the clock, developing manuals and marketing materials, camp sites, and a website. They decided on a name that felt both descriptive and limitless: Open Sky.

Open Sky accepted its first student in May of 2006 and continues today as strong and vibrant as ever. Food continues to be a core component of the program's medicine, and has expanded to include vegetables grown year round in Open Sky's own greenhouse dome. Yoga and meditation are daily program practices. The program's psychiatrist has weekly contact with students both in and out of the field. Every month since the first summer, parents have travelled to Durango for the Parent Wellness Weekend, not to see their children but to support them by doing their own work. Hundreds of families have gone through 3-day Family Quests.

The values that drove Open Sky from the beginning are still those that drive the program today. The learning and growing never stops, and the answer to Aaron's original question, "Are you still in?," is a resounding yes for Open Sky.

Chapter 20

Aspiro Adventure, est. April 1, 2006

Jess Shade

https://aspiroadventure.com

IN EARLY 2006, SEVERAL MINDS GOT TOGETHER TO answer the question, "How can we better engage our students in therapy and facilitate lasting change?" Initially answering this question in the context of a small residential treatment center, Aspiro began leading adventure activities to enhance the therapeutic experience of students. Blending front-country experiences (i.e., resort skiing, mountain biking, day hiking in Arches and Canyonlands National Parks, etc.) with the traditional remoteness of backcountry settings, the Aspiro team set out to challenge the notion that desert asceticism was the best or only way to reach struggling teenagers and young adults within the field of wilderness therapy. With Brian Church, Josh Watson, Justin Robinson, Randy Oakley, Farrah Jensen, Dave Ward, and Dan Lemaire, the Aspiro Adventure team began to take shape and broke away from the residential facility. Brian came from a family background of therapeutic programs and lent his expertise to structuring the young company and to marketing the new concepts. Josh, Justin, and Farrah all had therapeutic licenses and experience in wilderness or experiential education settings. Justin became the first clinical director while Josh who possessed the gift of communicating with families in crisis during their initial contact call, became the leader of the admissions team. Randy Oakley, Aspiro's first program director, employed his background in experiential education and therapeutic boarding schools by creating adventure sequencing with therapeutic intent. Due to his experience with recreational therapy, Dave orchestrated logistics, itineraries, and training. Dan, a passionate athlete and adventurer, structured the on-the-ground expeditions, sequencing, and therapeutic framework for each day. The program took shape on the banks of the Duchesne River in the Uinta Mountains at a small basecamp with one therapist, four guides, one female student, and a lot of heart.

The inspiration for Aspiro found its genesis in the desire to match or exceed the metaphoric capability of the primitive wilderness therapy model. With adventure activities to which students, their parents, and their home communities could relate, Aspiro sought to explore the deeper applications of drive, desire, and tolerance for adversity. These, the founders concluded, would provide the building blocks of therapeutic change that was lasting and directly applicable to the challenges inherent in life. By removing students from standard clinical settings and eliciting direct engagement with adventure activities, students would no longer be able to use the trite and empty "therapy speech." Instead, by living and overcoming challenges which were both novel and fully committing, students would experience therapeutic growth directly. Solely talking about therapeutic change proved much less effective than truly living and practicing the concepts each day in these varied challenging settings. Processing these experiences and debriefing challenges provided case studies in the true stuff of life with which students were dealing...or had been avoiding.

To achieve this therapeutic setting for grappling with challenges directly and practicing an empowered acceptance of change, Aspiro established a relational approach to therapy founded on the tenets of positive psychology. Strengths-based interventions focused through the lens of adventure activities were a new proving ground for Aspiro's foundational theory that self-efficacy is generalizable and critical in creating lasting therapeutic change. Field guides and therapists sought to increase buy-in from the students, allowing them to claim agency over their own therapeutic growth and the trajectory of their lives. By offering diverse adventures such as rock climbing, canyoneering, mountain biking, skiing, and backpacking, students could explore a variety of contexts in which they could set relevant new goals, challenge themselves within a group context, and experience overwhelming mastery experiences (OMEs). OMEs occur when a person chooses to undertake a challenge that is outside of their "comfort zone" and near the outside edge of their "learning zone." Assessing risk, capability, personal history, and desire, field guides do not assign or fabricate OME moments, but rather encourage and coach participants to be the engineers of their own successes. Managing one's fear, excitement, doubts, and other emotions to undertake a personal challenge allows the student to not only feel successful, but to self-identify as a capable individual. The capability to "work a climbing route" many times and ultimately reach the summit transfers directly into student beliefs that they can achieve challenging goals in life. OMEs remain an integral part of Aspiro's culture today.

Engaging therapeutic change with the students provided much of the drive for creating a new adventure-based model. Additionally, anticipating expectations from the parents provided the impetus for other important deviations from the traditional wilderness therapy model. Weekly showers, a family seminar in the middle of the student's stay and (privately) posted numerous weekly pictures of the student were all aspects added early on in Aspiro's history. A basecamp model became a central piece of logistics to allow for more formal therapy time and the opportunity to travel to new course areas each week. Parents used the adventure activities and the photos from all over the state of Utah as a way of sharing their child's experiences with their larger circles of family and friends. The guilt and shame of seeking treatment for their adolescent and young adult children were lessened by bridges to adventure experiences that were relatable. Parents wanted to tell others about their child's successes in learning to climb, bike, ski, and camp.

Today, Aspiro maintains diverse groups year-round with exceptional clinicians and a large contingent of guides to meet each student's needs. Therapists have the ability to add evidence-based specialized programming for their group, such as allowing a young adult group to practice the 12-Step Model and attend AA meetings. Cognitive Behavior Therapy (CBT) remains integral for the "quirky" groups whereas Dialectical Behavior Therapy (DBT) is the primary model for adolescent girls who struggle with abuse, personality disorders, and behavioral challenges. Additionally, the goal of best serving these students is met through programmatic flexibility, with choice between diverse geographic locations, adventure activities, and front-country versus back-country exposure rates. These factors allow for a wide range of experiences in which guides and clinicians can assess their students. Students who are entrenched in certain behaviors or cognitive distortions are continually encouraged to reset their experience by being in a novel and varied environment each week. Every week clinicians, guides, and field management exchange ideas about what itinerary will be of the most value to the students in each of their groups.

Integral to Aspiro's early and continued success has been a focus on best practices within the industry fueled by ongoing research efforts. Partnering with Dr. Mark Widmer of BYU, Aspiro has run ongoing studies with students while they were attending Aspiro and beyond. Focus groups of guides, clinicians, and management members have provided valuable sources of feedback via consistent self-audits. The common desire is to build and re-build the Aspiro model around the best evidence, to constantly adapt as new information emerges, approach our own practices with a healthy skepticism, to question much more, and regularly.

Today the guiding principles of creating challenging, novel, and transferable experiential therapy remain at the core of Aspiro. Agency, solution-focused thinking, and strengths-based goal setting continue to inspire students toward lasting therapeutic change. In keeping with the focus on research, innovation, and flexibility, Aspiro continues to add new elements to the program. Constantly questioning, the Aspiro team asked, "can our students graduate feeling more confident in succeeding academically and possess more interest in engaging in lifelong learning?" In response, Aspiro totally revamped the academic curriculum to allow for increased flexibility across different ages and academic focal points of its diverse student body. With an eye on risk management data collected internally and industry-wide, Aspiro asked, "how do we add to the physical safety of our adventures while getting even deeper with their therapeutic elements?" In response, an entire team was dedicated for adventure facilitation trainings which now occur on a weekly basis with a focus not only on the hard skills of each adventure, but also on sequencing for therapeutic intent. As a leader in the adventure therapy industry, Aspiro's conference sponsorship and attendance, independent workshops for professionals, and alumni outreach events continue to grow in quantity and quality each year. Having served over 3,500 students since 2006, Aspiro possesses a depth of experiential knowledge within the field of adventure therapy and continues to be a frontrunner of new and exciting innovations. For example, in 2013 Pure Life opened in Costa Rica as a young adult therapeutic transitional living program, making Aspiro the first wilderness therapy program to develop an international treatment option. It is truly an exciting time to be a part of this company and to be a part of the larger wilderness adventure therapy field. Aspiro's definition "to ascend, to aspire, to infuse spirit" remains a vibrant response to a world in need.

Chapter 21

2007: Story of New Vision Wilderness History

Drew Hornbeck and Steve Sawyer, Co-Founders

http://newvisionwilderness.com

BEFORE NEW VISION WILDERNESS – DREW: ON A summer camp canoe trip in northern Wisconsin as a 10 year old boy, I had a formative experience. We had two canoes; one occupied by me (in the stern) and 2 other boys, and the other with the trip leader and a camper. The trip leader's canoe went much faster and eventually the canoe I was in fell far behind. As we came to a fork in the river and our calls for help went unanswered, the boys in my canoe became nervous. One boy started crying and the other was shutting down into a quiet panic. I knew something had to be done, so I decided it would be best to turn the boat around and head back up river returning to the put-in, rather than risk taking a wrong fork in the river and getting lost with a group of scared boys.

I thought little of this experience until my mid-30's when I became the founder/co-owner of 2 wilderness therapy programs. I realized more than 20 years later that the experience in the canoe was the first decision I had made as an outdoor leader!

From the Clinic to the Woods – Steve: After 10 years of intensive work in an office setting, more time in the outdoors was very appealing. The raw wilderness had been my healer in other stages of life, and I knew it could help others in the same way.

I had been seeing clients in the office for many sessions but when they attended clinically intensive retreats in the outdoors, they began to make big strides during those breaks from the "plastic" world. I was mesmerized by the shift that occurred in clients as they were entranced by the flames of a fire and by the stars flickering in the late night sky. Treatment just simply moved faster outdoors.

As time went on, I preferred to grab my rig (packed backpack) over my briefcase and I desired more of these rapid clinical results. When Drew and I met, the appeal of full blown immersed expeditions over short-term retreats was an easy decision. There was an additional energetic gain that seemed to increase my clinical endurance. The work in the woods felt beautiful. As our systems began to dial in, the strategic use of exercise, relational immersion, and clinical timing all began to increase the results. Kids who had been virtually unreachable suddenly became reachable.

Partnership – Drew: In early 2007 I received a call from NVW's Northern Wisconsin field area. It was Steve, my new business partner. He launched into this story, "From across the pond we heard yells and screams of joy from our group of teenage boys and staff. I'm telling you I didn't think they would find one! Now what are we going to do?" Steve went on to explain the outcome of an exercise on "find your survival food," of which very few were ever successful – until now. Steve had told the boys if they caught a frog he would let them try frog legs for the first time. *They caught a frog.* Steve led the group in a ceremony for the frog, teaching them to respect wildlife. And then they tried frog legs for the first time. Since those early days of NVW, other than fish, no other animals have been killed in our program!

Prior to the frog hunt, Steve and I had been operating our own small weekend camping excursions independently with the goal of helping young men learn more about themselves and our natural environment. We didn't know each other, but we had been doing very similar work. When a colleague introduced us for the first time, it was evident immediately that if we combined our strengths, mine in outdoor programming, risk management, and relational approach and Steve's expertise in clinical models and intervention that we had something special.

Clinical Model Development – Drew and Steve: We agreed from the beginning that wilderness therapy should be based in Trauma Informed Care, relational-approach, and customized to the individual. In 2008 NVW started running 21-day programs and continued that model for

5 years. We were fortunate to hire some dynamic and passionate leaders who are still with us today.

In 2011 NVW launched Quest, our program providing clients longer term treatment than the initial 21 day model. We purchased a beautiful 40 acres adjacent to our field area and moved operations into the NVW Lodge. That year NVW adopted the Mastery system. Mastery sets aside level and phases, rather the client has a choice to learn what they want to become the master of, where choice is a dictating variable for the individual. This supports igniting or relighting a spark within and allows the individual to buy-in to the program.

Clinical immersion is a key variable at New Vision Wilderness and presence during therapeutic windows is critical to the NVW model. NVW's trained and certified therapists work in the woods 3 days a week, living side-by-side with clients. Other therapeutic modalities such as Heartmath, EMDR, Brainspotting, Art Therapy, and Trauma Sensitive Yoga are integrated and work in tandem with NVW's relational philosophies.

Expanding Out West – Drew and Steve: Having a history of working with young adults on individualized treks, in 2012 (with the help of experienced wilderness experts Rob Koning and Lonnie Drouhard), NVW launched its West Coast Young Adult Program in the Cascade Mountains. This customized approach to helping those aged 18-25 get back on their feet includes Life Opportunities for Transformation (LOFT), a transitional component providing opportunities for transitions and experiences in the community coupled with a return to their group in the woods for processing. LOFT includes outdoor adventures, community integration, and/or vocational work.

Not long after launching the Young Adult Program, NVW received an adolescent license through the state of Oregon to serve boys ages 13 to 17.

The Growth of our Adventure Model – Drew and Steve: Adventure education has always been integrated at NVW. We believe that providing peak experiences while pushing comfort zones and learning to trust others are key components toward creating safe and healthy relationships. NVW's Wisconsin location has a lengthy history of canoe and white water expeditions. Rock climbing, cross country skiing, fishing, and other adventure activities are also incorporated into NVW's programming.

In 2012 NVW joined OBH. We have been proud to join this group of professional people and support the development of outdoor behavioral healthcare as an effective, legitimate, and evidence-based option for families

Summary – Drew: NVW was born in the basement of my house in Milwaukee and our first trips were loaded into the back of a Subaru wagon. Steve was the therapist and I was the field staff. Now in 2015, NVW serves 180 adolescents and young adults annually and employs more than 70 full time people across 2 states.

NVW recently partnered with CALO, a residential program for adopted children run by a dedicated team of professionals. Both entities operate as individual programs, yet this exciting collaboration supports working together for program quality, research, and best practices for the youth of today and tomorrow.

Chapter 22

2008: Elements Wilderness Program

John Karren and Andrew Powell

http://www.elementswilderness.com

Iₙ May 2008, John Karren, Lynn Smith, and Karen Scrafford (formerly Hesselman) set out to create a small, hands-on, intimate wilderness program for boys. Seeing wilderness programs grow and become large corporations, they wanted to get back to the foundation of wilderness therapy and create a specific program that would resonate with boys and their families.

Lynn discovered Aspen Achievement Academy in 1994 and began work as a field staff. He moved to Second Nature in 1999 where he again worked as a field staff, and met John Karren. While there he earned his Master's degree in Social Work from the University of Utah and eventually became a therapist working with boys. Lynn was there for close to 10 years as a staff and therapist. It was during that transition from direct care staff to therapist that Lynn realized just how much he did not know all those years ago when he began working on the trail. This knowledge gap between the therapists who design the programs and the field staff who spend 99% of the time with the students had tremendous impact on Lynn and he carried that with him years later, as he set out to create Elements.

John started working at Second Nature in the admissions department. During his first week training in the field, he set out in an attempt to understand what wilderness was all about and to figure out why he would want to commit to such a strange endeavor. As it turns out, he was amazed to find himself in the middle of nowhere with great people, all of them facilitating incredible work in a group of tenacious and resilient boys.

Karen started as a field staff at the Duchesne location of Second Nature as well. She was graduating from college and looking for an outdoor job. She found several that were 20 day courses in the summer, but then she came across wilderness therapy. Still not knowing what she was getting into, she committed to a training and jumped in blind. She thought she would likely move on after two years, but that was in 2001. In the years that followed, Karen moved into field management, where she learned the need for consistency in a field where everything from weather to moods were constantly in flux.

In early 2008, John approached Lynn about doing something different as the program where they were working had grown exponentially into one of the largest in the country. They talked about getting back to their roots with an intentionally small program where they would know every family and individualize their treatment to match each family's needs. They talked about a program that gave staff and students the tools they needed to progress each week into deeper growth and understanding. They talked about finding new ways to make the most of the precious little window of time they are given with each student and family.

In thinking about someone to run the operations, Lynn said the only person he wanted was Karen, and that proved to be a key decision in the creation of the company as Karen agreed to become an owner and the Program Director. She joined the conversation and spoke of professionalism, consistency, and providing a solid model to all her staff so that each individual in the program knew how important they were to the whole.

It was in this vein that the three forged ahead as founders and owners of the new little company called Elements. Elements right from the start was packed with talent. They were approached by two friends that were coming out of graduate school with MSW's and were looking for jobs. Jen Rapp and Tara Stireman (formerly Feeney) came onboard as the first set of field mentors. Tara and Jen later took command of their own groups, and Tara is still with Elements today.

As the company expanded, Neal Christensen, Ph.D and Andrew Powell were brought on as partners as well, to help Elements move beyond "startup mode" and into a sustainable future serving our students and families. Elements has always been committed and remains committed to being truly "owner operated." As John puts it, "I think at some point we all looked up from running this thing for seven years and said, 'I don't think we can continue like this for seven more years.'" Andrew became the Executive Director, where he helps each department perform at its highest capability, and Neal took his seat as Elements' first psychologist, working with his own group of boys and strengthening the core of the clinical team.

As we continued to integrate our clinical work into the field operations of our program, we have been fortunate to add a unique adventure program. These adventure activities are accomplished by groups hiking to and from the adventure sites while remaining in-line with their constant expedition itineraries. We see this as critical as it allows the treatment process to continue without interruption. Karen carries her commitment to each individual in our program to heart. Karen has a strong work ethic and pours that care and concern into every bit of the operation of Elements. This ranges to all students, staff, employees, and the everyday job.

In creating Elements, John found a place that he could do his job to his own high standards, connecting with families and truly knowing all within his program. He remains the first voice at the other end of the line when a family calls the admissions line, and there is nothing more satisfying in his career than the deep connections he's made with all the other people in this field who have the same heart he does for our kids.

From the start, Lynn has taken a vital part in the inception of the program and provided clinical vision. Being a Clinical Social Worker with over a decade of experience as a Field Staff, Lynn has a profound understanding of wilderness and the metaphors it offers. He built the clinical foundation, and more than that, he wove it into the daily life and jobs of our field mentors from their first day on the trail. It is there that Lynn has brought the best of evidence-based practice into balance with the pragmatic lessons and metaphors that can only be found while living in the middle of the wilderness with a group of teenaged boys.

Elements is unique in the synergy between the clinical and the field departments. What we find most critical in our culture is that no one believes they personally hold all the answers as to what specifically makes our 8-10 week program work. This we believe will keep us keen-eyed and ready to continue to adapt and grow into a program that will serve boys in the best way we can, with these precious little windows of time we have available to us.

The summer of 2015 has just ended and Elements has just finished its 8th summer in operation. It has been an amazing journey, we have grown closer as a partnership and it truly feels like we are the Elements family. It hasn't been easy, as we started in 2008, which will go down in history as one of the most difficult financial times for our country as well as this industry. It was a challenging period to endure. We have experienced some of the greatest moments of our lives, and of course had some very tough moments and decisions to be made. The one thing we can say about Elements is that we all recognize that it is in the whole that each of us as individuals find our strength. Not one of us puts our self ahead of the company or makes decisions based on finances alone; Elements was founded on and continues to be a student-first mentality, and one that we hope will have the great fortune to serve many more families for years to come.

Chapter 23

2008: History of WinGate

Shayne Gallagher

http://www.wingatewildernesstherapy.com

THE FOUNDING OF WINGATE WILDERNESS THERAPY is based on its people and their histories, the nature of it' location, and it's principles of operation.

The Northern Arizona/Southern Utah high desert is, in my mind and heart, a magical and mystical place. It is vast, open, and visually far reaching; one's senses can take in a swath of a thousand square miles of nearly uninhabited terrain…from standing almost anywhere in its "Great Circle." It is peppered by only a few small towns, one of which I grew up in.

This desert contains striking contrast, inviting full attention to that which sustains beings existing within it. Where it is dry…it is bone dry. Yet scattered about, as though strategically, are water stores and springs, evidencing in their vicinity, generation's worth of living and thriving. On most given days, but especially on a brisk winter's morning, the boundary of the difference in temperature, from shade to sun, is itself palpable. Many of the desert's endemic plants are rugged, sharp, and scratchy, and yet, just over a barren red dirt bank…down in the creek's mini-green-belt-valley-way, abounds hanging gardens, green leafy edible treasures, and huge trees that pump hundreds of gallons of water per day into a thirsty turquoise sky. It is an ancient and current sacred ground for many overlapping indigenous and colonizing peoples from several eras.... It has also been sacred ground for me.

Growing up in a difficult and confusing home life, my soul longed for solace, and...looking back on it, a permanence that "stable unchanging things" seemed to somehow be able to provide. Behind my house, up the hill, surrounded by medium sized green-blue juniper trees, various lizards and an occasional rattlesnake, was a Mogollon Culture ruin. Digging around in the sand, collecting yards of pottery, hunting horned toads, and simply being alone amongst all of the desert things, was for me, in a word...safe. I could (and often would) escape to a nearby canyon, and spend many contiguous hours alone, wondering after the petroglyphs left by ancient mysterious forerunners, who must of known, well, something I didn't...something from their time and place, and they left their mark of it...on stone...and in my heart's imagination...sometimes I wonder if, during times like those, I was really alone.

When I was fourteen, on a Sunday morning, I was informed that my father had passed away during the night. As surprise, confusion and pain seared through my mind, the first thing I thought to do was to run to my desert place. I sat at the base of one of my friends, one of the green-blue junipers, for the better part of that day....

Years later I was introduced to a man by the name of Larry Olson. He had recently started a "Wilderness Survival Program" for teenagers. They needed young people as staff, and I needed a job. My first few days in the field could best be described (by me at the time) as tormenting. Sure I loved the desert, but in all my previous experiences I had always taken along food that I liked, soda pop I enjoyed, and anything else I thought I needed...including matches. Plus I had never spent so many days in a row away from some sort of access to a bathroom. I had decided that anyone who does this for a living has got to either be a masochist, insane, or just plain stupid. During those first few days, if there had been a way out, I would have taken it. Then, in the middle of the night, after an agonizingly long hike, one of the boys in the group asked me, *"So have you decided if you are going to work here?"* The question cut just a little, because I had decided that I was absolutely not going to work there, but I didn't want to make him feel bad so I responded, *"I haven't decided yet."* Then he asked me, *"Do you think you could at least work here until I leave?"* When one allows one's heart to be touched, difficulties of circumstances gain a new perspective. I couldn't ignore his request. I stayed until that young man left…and, in wilderness therapy…twenty-five more years.

During her college career, Sheri was mentored by some of the pioneers of both wilderness survival and wilderness therapy, perhaps most notably Doug Nelson, who trusted Sheri to teach his recreation and survival courses, and who then asked Sheri to develop aspects of the first long term (meaning longer than three weeks) wilderness therapy program he was designing. She did so. Sheri was the first female senior staff of the first long-term wilderness therapy program in the industry. A couple of years or so later, she shifted gears and went to work for another wilderness program, which is where I had been working for a couple of months. We were married six months later.

Sheri and I have worked on a number of wilderness therapy related projects and programs over the years. During part of that time she took a long break from directly working with programs, in order to raise our six children, all of whom, at this point have now worked in a wilderness therapy job of one kind or another themselves.

We were both working in yet another wilderness therapy program when a man who possesses a keen entrepreneurial spirit approached us. His proposal was simple: *"You know how to design and operate a wilderness therapy program, and I know how to fund the starting of a program, and how to run several aspects of the business side of it. We are all partners and co-owners. What do you think?"* It did not take much convincing. 18 years of designing and helping operate other people's programs seemed like quality preparation to start our own. The offer seemed, and more importantly felt, both right and timely. Tim Dupell continues to be our partner, friend, mentor, and "investor" in untold ways.

Few therapists have the unique combination of clinical expertise, extreme amount of experience in the field, and distinctive ability to "let the wilderness be the therapist" as Scott Hess. Sheri and I had gotten to know Scott over the preceding two years, working together and gaining an understanding of each other's approach to working with young people. In a very short period of time, we knew that Scott's approach to working with children matched ours in profound ways. When Scott found out we were starting a new program, he wanted to be part of it, and we were glad he did.

Some people have a natural, unforced way of communicating that makes others feel immediately comfortable and understood. This ability is, in my opinion, less of an acquired talent and more of an innate characteristic. This characteristic requires genuine caring for the person they are talking to. Brad Matheson is one of those people. Sheri and I had worked in a program together with Brad several years earlier, and heard through the grapevine that he might be available for a proposal. I literally drove around his neighborhood, trying to remember where he lived.... I found him.

"Wingate" is the name of one of the many layers of sandstone found in the canyons and rock formations of Northern Arizona and Southern Utah. It occurs in the general area where WinGate Wilderness Therapy operates. It is recognizable for It's red, solid, tall cliff face features. Sheri, Scott, Brad, and I, from the beginning, have shared a clear understanding of the principles we believe should be the bedrock of any wilderness therapy program, and have endeavored to follow those from day one of the inception of WinGate.

Some of those principles include the importance of teaching solid principles on a daily basis, the treating of students with absolute respect, with the idea that we are all of great worth, and that students have just as much to give, share, and as do the staff who care for them, that program personnel must learn how to behave in order to be chosen as a mentor, and that the wilderness has its own amazing gifts to give, lessons to provide, and healing power to impart. To the degree we can reach into it, without interruption, is the degree to which it can distill upon us, that which is there to receive.

There were several others present at the inception of WinGate who played important roles in it's realization, and others who have joined it's ranks as partners who add inestimable value to it's success, notably Greg Hitchcock, who's character and work ethic are inestimable. They all left their "mark of it" and continue to leave their mark on it...they have placed their own petroglyphs on the WinGate cliff face wall.

Chapter 24

2008: Trails Carolina History

Brian Johnson

http://trailscarolina.com

T HE INAUGURAL GROUP OF STUDENTS AT TRAILS Carolina had just completed its first wilderness expedition and returned to base camp to celebrate the accomplishment. It was Thanksgiving, 2008, and the five adolescent girls that made up the group had bonded over the course of their two weeks on the trail. Together they had endured the elements, the hiking and the inevitable conflict that arises as a result of communal living. Their group had come out of the woods as a highly functional team, excited and proud to have shared the experience.

Shalene Pierce, one of the founding members of Trails Carolina, was the primary therapist for that first group of students. At the start of Trails, Shalene had over a decade of experience in wilderness therapy, pulling insight from an internship at Second Nature, several years at SUWS of the Carolinas, and a 6-month stint at Adirondack Leadership Expeditions, where the New England cold drove this Texas-raised therapist back to more southern climes. It was her work in southern Appalachia that made her nationally renowned within the industry for her success with adolescent girls facing a myriad of struggles, particularly trauma.

Shalene's group of five girls had shared a peak experience recognizable to anyone familiar with the field of wilderness therapy. The girls were happy, excited, and functional. And, as many parents who have sent their child to wilderness would know, the honeymoon doesn't last.

Barely 30 minutes had passed since the girls had returned from their expedition, and the group was falling apart. The social and emotional skills learned on the trail appeared to have vanished as soon as the girls were back on familiar ground. Shalene, confused and frustrated by the group having taken two steps back, sought out Trails Carolina's founder and Executive Director, Graham Shannonhouse, to voice her concerns.

In return, Graham smiled, pointed to the group, and reassuringly reminded Shalene, "This is exactly what we wanted."

Graham Shannonhouse is an unassuming and introverted leader. Though she has been in the industry for over 20 years she still exhibits a fierce passion for the work. Even now she draws upon her time as field staff, artfully crafting stories of her own successes and failures so to teach the lessons-learned to a new generation of wilderness therapy employees.

Graham was introduced to wilderness therapy in 1994 as a field instructor, leading 3-week expeditions in the desert of southern Idaho. After 2 years, she became a field supervisor, and in 1998 she developed and ran the first wilderness therapy youth program in the nation. In 2002 Graham was transferred from Idaho to help resurrect a struggling SUWS of the Carolinas, where she served as the Executive Director for 6 years before opening Trails Carolina in 2008.

A lifetime career in the industry had given Graham time to dream of what she'd do differently if given the opportunity to start her own program. Two clear goals she had for Trails were to create an empowering wilderness expedition model that regularly brought students out of the woods to intentionally practice transition skills, and to create a program that truly addressed the family component instead of only treating the "identified patient." Graham herself is fond of saying, "We've taken this really simple idea of wilderness therapy and made it really complicated." Indeed, Graham's vision to deeply integrate these two pillars into a wilderness therapy model proved to be a challenge, but they are also what set Trails Carolina apart from its peers.

The group of girls that fell apart within 30 minutes of returning from their wilderness expedition had proven a point: the lessons from the trail are not seamlessly transferable to a more normal ("real world") setting. The base camp and classroom components of the Trails expedition model of wilderness therapy stand to contextualize the lessons learned on the trail. Cabins, chores, school, extracurriculars, and homework all invite the student to practice transitioning out of the woods, while still benefitting from the support systems of the program.

The move from a purely nomadic model to one in which the expedition is periodically punctuated with stays on campus was, and still is, a teachable moment for the program. The development of meaningful basecamp programming and the logistical demands of a program with so many moving parts continues to be a balancing act between efficiency, customer service, and therapeutic "mile-posting."

In opening Trails Carolina, Graham also sought to revolutionize how wilderness therapy addresses not just the child in the woods, but the entire family system. Since the onset, intentional family programming integrated into treatment has been the gold standard of Trails Carolina. In fact, Trails was a pioneer in hiring a designated family therapist. And while the list of family services has only grown since 2008, the program has succeeded in not treating them as mere add-ons to the child's work, but instead are integral pieces of the treatment and transition plans.

The history of Trails Carolina has been one of finding the right people to successfully pull together the components of wilderness expedition, base camp programming, and integrated family work into one cohesive service. One of Graham's favorite leadership analogies comes from Jim Collins' book, *Good to Great: Why Some Companies Make the Leap… and Others Don't,* in which the author explains that a company must first seek to "get the right people on the bus" and then get everyone sitting in the right place.

Graham remembers that it took 3-4 years to get people in the right seats on the bus and establish a cohesive team ready to do the work. It was around then that the clinical staff, as a group, started to come of age. In addition, Graham found the right people to start developing the basecamp programming into something more structured and meaningful. Also around that time, the abrupt departure of an administrator kick-started a tough year for Trails. But the setback strengthened the resolve of the program and launched a continuing period of growth for Trails.

One of Trails Carolina's greatest successes has been in assembling a highly skilled team that is passionate about the benefits of wilderness therapy delivered to its students and families when wilderness expeditions are, at the core, integrated with meaningful basecamp programming and a comprehensive family approach.

Chapter 25

2010: History Of Expedition Therapy

Beth Fogel

http://expeditiontherapy.com

EXPEDITION THERAPY OPENED ITS DOORS IN OCTOBER 2010 as a structured, intensive, hands-on, experiential, solution-focused experience for emerging young adults age 18+ who have yet to find a productive and intentional path in life. Beginning with two field areas, Expedition Therapy created Canyoneering, Backpacking, and Rock Climbing Expeditions.

The Expedition Therapy outdoor adventure experience therapeutic curriculum was created by Beth J. Fogel, MSW, CSW, who had worked as a primary therapist in a variety of wilderness settings. She came to realize that there were no real options for emerging adults needing to connect with their true potential, discover their unique direction in life, and take their places in the adult world with confidence and purpose.

Having seen the limitations of existing young adult wilderness programs that were much the same as their adolescent counterparts, Beth had a vision of a unique, experiential, hands-on approach that would meet the very specific needs young adults having difficulty transitioning into adult life, or who struggle with specific issues such as alternative learning styles, ADD, school failure, lack of motivation, depression and social anxiety. Her brilliant idea was to use outdoor experiential activities that require professional hands-on training, in conjunction with a thoroughly integrated therapeutic culture, to help these young adults launch into their lives.

Beth originated Expedition Therapy as a series of challenging weekly expeditions, built around her innovative Therapeutic Expedition Mentality®, a very sophisticated hands-on clinical and experiential approach to leadership, personal growth, and empowerment for young adults. Using an all-inclusive approach, Expedition Therapy Field Instructors of all levels work in tandem with Therapists as a team, emphasizing a strengths and empowerment perspective to relate to and connect with students who are at the beginning of their adult lives. The Expedition Therapy team's initial focus with students is upon relationship building, taking the necessary time for students to acclimate to our various environments, and to work on honing their communication skills. Over a period of eight to twelve weeks, relationships become strengthened, confidence is restored, and an awareness of new ways of coping and effective problem-solving evolves. Expedition Therapy's relationship based model has, as its centerpiece, engagement, trust, respect, and unconditional positive regard. Students experience many successes each day, whether learning safety protocols, single pitch climbing, or mediating a relevant group topic with their peers.

It took a skilled, integrated team to bring Expedition Therapy into existence as an experience that provides participants with individualized therapy in the context of a back country skills and leadership course. Aaron Wilson, who holds a B.S. in Outdoor Recreation Management with an emphasis in Experiential Education and is also a Certified PCS Trainer, led the field staff. Wes Light, a Wilderness EMT who is also a WEA National Standards Program Instructor, oversaw the weekly expedition curriculum and the permits for the field areas that have increased to the current eight that the company operates in. The wide variety of field areas was chosen to provide multiple expedition options that include rock climbing, canyoneering, cultural exploration, mountaineering, backpacking, kayaking and more.

High standards were established for field staff, requiring college degrees, personal maturity, WFR certifications, and a hard-to-find combination of outdoor technical expertise combined with therapeutic relational and processing skills. Expedition Therapy Field Instructors are teachers, mentors and therapeutic facilitators during each week's expedition and at base camp. In conjunction with a highly qualified clinical staff, deeply experienced in outdoor behavioral health care, Expedition Therapy achieved excellent outcomes for most students right from the start. A commitment was made from day one that no matter what approaches were used, the individual students' outcomes would be priority one.

Our first student was a young man who made a tough but amazing journey from a very dark place to a bright future. We were privileged to accompany him and facilitate his progress. Many others have followed in his footsteps, discovering that they too can emerge as their best selves and take charge of their lives.

Safety has been our top priority since the inception. Expedition Therapy offers students the safest and highest quality wilderness therapy and outdoor leadership training available. Risk management and incident response training are included in all of our courses. Our excellent safety record is a function of this as well as the professionalism, emergency response experience and competency of our staff.

Since those early days, the Expedition Therapy curriculum has constantly evolved to meet the needs of our students and their families. In addition to the original weekly expeditions, we have added service-oriented front country expeditions at an animal sanctuary, at community events and in the National Parks. These experiences build character and an understanding of "giving back," providing each student with opportunities to practice skills in the world, in real time, and in community settings.

Expedition Therapy has also incorporated a variety of certification courses for students, including Wilderness Advanced First Aid, SCUBA, and Avalanche Safety. These hands-on courses teach valuable skills that can be used for a lifetime. Our unique "Take Flight" expedition teaches students the skills needed to build and fly model airplanes, as a metaphor for launching into life. We take into account each student's individual interests and are consistently adding new expeditions so students can reconnect with passions they may have abandoned because of their personal difficulties.

To improve our students' family systems, Expedition Therapy introduced Family Expeditions, which bring together the Expedition Therapy student and his or her closest family members, providing an opportunity to resolve relationship-based issues and reconnect in a positive way.

We at Expedition Therapy are proud of our ability to be powerful catalysts in the personal growth process between students and their families. Our commitment to being "change agents" in the lives of our students and their families is evidenced by a large percentage of successful outcomes in the past four years. Students who successfully complete Expedition Therapy move forward more confidently, with more motivation and with a strengthened family structure, well-prepared to take their places in adult society. We will continue to empower each student to identify his or her passions, interests and needs, intensively mentor them and create a supportive space where they can experience many successes every day.

Chapter 26

2010: Adventure Works

Lynette Spencer

http://www.adventureworksdekalb.org

As a social worker in the behavioral health field, MY earlier years were spent working behind locked doors and sealed windows – on an inpatient psychiatric unit, accompanied by twenty-four hour emergency department crisis assessment responsibilities. Later on, I found my way into a well-appointed office at the multi-specialty DeKalb Clinic. I paid my dues and was now in private practice, setting my own (daytime) hours, and seeing patients who were *voluntarily* seeking help. The downside of private practice was the sedentary nature of the job and rather than windows that didn't open, I simply had no window. Even more concerning was the population who were no longer my clients: the poor. Poverty doesn't equal mental illness, but surely creates a risk factor, and for children, a much higher risk of trauma exposure. Poverty is not just a paucity of finances, but of positive experiences as well.

Somewhere in the mid-1990's while still working with inpatient behavioral health, I came to know a fellow social worker who seemed to help solve all of my "placement problems," otherwise known as patients, who had nowhere to go upon discharge. Lesly Wicks, LCSW, Executive Director of Hope Haven Homeless Shelter, has a passion for homelessness and needs of the poor. Lesly became a trusted colleague and friend who shared my vision for something more than the traditional route to wellness. Some fifteen years later, she and I became the co-founders of Adventure Works.

Around the same time I met Lesly, a psychiatrist gave me an article about equine assisted psychotherapy (EAP). This writing resonated with me as I had recently become a horse owner and thought it the perfect marriage between two of my passions. In 2002, my first horse Bailey (a beautifully strong, sixteen hand, dark bay Thoroughbred) was diagnosed with West Nile Virus, even after being vaccinated. After a year of challenges, it became clear that her balance would not be restored for riding and I would need to find her a different purpose. After a Google search and a few phone calls, I came into contact with a small Elburn, Illinois program called Harnessing Hope; the owner had no need for a horse but the therapist in her program had just gone on maternity leave. After one phone conversation and a meeting at Starbucks, I was on my way to Jacksonville, Florida for my first EAP certification training (EAGALA model) and was practicing EAP with a few of my private practice patients just two months thereafter. What? I could wear jeans to "work" and be in the majestic presence of horses, all within the realm of my social work career? I didn't look back. My office-based talk therapy practice became secondary and I saw clients grow and change more efficiently than ever in the indoor arena. I was hooked, and talking about it to anyone who would listen.

Lesly listened, and began writing grants so her clients could benefit as well. She wrote two successful grants that funded three programs: equine assisted youth group, equine assisted parenting group, and a collaborative equine assisted youth camp that served homeless and domestic violence sheltered youth one summer. The success of these three programs over the course of two years (2006-7) sparked discussion of a "working farm" – one that would give homeless people a sense of purpose giving back to the community in which they lived, whether it be through the vegetable crops raised or the wool sheared from the flock of sheep they tended.

In the fall of 2009 I was teaching as an adjunct faculty member at Aurora University. Due to my equine work I was asked to teach a new elective course, offered in the child welfare track of the MSW program, on expressive and experiential therapy. The goal of this course was to introduce students to alternative ways to reach children in counseling. Throughout that semester, I used guest speakers and field trips to teach this course through experiential learning. One guest session, taught by Chicago Adventure Therapy, introduced me to what I now know as the umbrella model of Adventure Therapy upon which Adventure Works is based. Little did I know that EAP was just one of many forms of adventure therapy, alongside hiking, paddling, climbing, and many other outdoor sports that are used in mental health treatment. Through this connection I was introduced to the greater community of the Therapeutic Adventure Professionals Group, associated with the Association of Experiential Education; I now serve as Treasurer of the TAPG Leadership Council and have gained immense knowledge and support from this group.

The core concept of the organization came by way of a challenge from a very practical student: Zimbawe Armstrong. Z, as she is called, astutely pointed out to me (several times) that learning these modalities were useless because the kids she and her classmates would be working with could not afford such specialty services (and State of Illinois funding certainly wouldn't pay for it). It was true: the experiential therapy modalities are prohibitively expensive, and are not covered by Medicaid. I had a quandary to confront: how to embrace the work I love and know to be effective, while making sure it is accessible to everyone.

Enter again Lesly, along with her MSW intern Ade Willrett, and coffee at Panera. My class was over in November 2009, and in December we made Panera our office. Multiple meetings over a few weeks' time led us to the conclusion that I would submit a grant to start a nonprofit adventure therapy agency for homeless youth and the DeKalb County Community Mental Health Board was identified as the funding source. The funding was submitted in February and fully approved three months later; we incorporated with the State of Illinois in May, formed a board of directors, and started Adventure Works: a nonprofit, outpatient, outdoor behavioral healthcare, groups-based adventure therapy organization, with a straight-forward mission: *"to assist youth in overcoming challenges and becoming healthy adults through adventure-based counseling."* The ideas suddenly became a reality and our first program was "off the ground" in November 2010 with my endlessly supportive husband, Don Spencer, as my volunteer co-facilitator: six homeless teenagers met over the course of four weekends, culminating their experience at the Outdoor Wisconsin Leadership School (OWLS) high ropes course on a snowy Saturday.

As I tell this story just five years after that first cup of coffee at Panera, I am humbled by Adventure Works' growth: We are serving more than one-hundred fifty youth per year and continuing to prioritize those living in poverty and homelessness by providing free services, and free transportation. Adventure therapy groups run six days per week, serving ages six through eighteen and provide transportation for about eighty percent of our youth. We have superb partnerships with our local forest preserves, parks, and archery club. This community-based agency is thriving through community-based relationships. Adventure Works has an eighty-eight percent attendance rate and promising outcomes, which are now being formalized with the Outdoor Behavioral Healthcare Research Cooperative (obhrc.org), to demonstrate that the Adventure Works community-based outdoor behavioral healthcare adventure therapy model is the right approach for reaching and creating positive change in kids. Our operating budget has gone from $35,595 to nearly $270,000, a board of three friends we cajoled has grown to an eleven member, professionally diverse, active and wonderfully supportive board of directors, and after two years of being the only employee, I now have a team of eight full and part time staff as well as five contracted staff. This month marks the inaugural planning of our adventure center, which will include that working farm Lesly and I dreamed about nearly twenty years ago.

Chapter 27

2012: The Journey, LLC and 1989 The Achievement Foundation: Wilderness Academy

Madolyn M. Liebing, Ph.D., Psychologist & LMFT

http://journeywilderness.com

"**H**OW CAN TAKING KIDS OUT OF CLASS TO GO hiking keep them from dropping out of high school?" The year was 1978, and the question was posed by our principal. Feeling like kids being called on the carpet ourselves, Gary Weaver and I sort of ducked our heads and searched for a way to answer this no-nonsense, suit and tie administrator.

"Well," Gary responded, rubbing his chin and looking for the right words, "most kids drop out because they are continually failing in school. Then they begin to feel like failures themselves and would rather avoid the place where they keep failing. With the trips we are planning, kids will have to work hard, but we can insure their success as long they put in some effort. They come out realizing that they can overcome hard things and school is one of the hard things they can do."

The principal looked skeptical. "And you can get this by hiking around in the desert? Aren't you rewarding them for not doing well? And why bring regular students with them?"

Thus began my life-long effort to convince people of the power of wilderness experiences. It was an uphill battle, but in the end, Gary (the school psychologist) and I (the high school counselor at the time) were able to organize and conduct short (six day) treks in the Southern Utah Desert. We called them Survival Trips, but they were really just backpacking trips with a 24-hour solo. The students brought their own equipment (we gave them a list) and paid $40 for food. The school district furnished a van and gas and our salaries. We would post a sign-up sheet in the spring and fall and usually by the end of the day, we would have 30 kids signed up and ready to go. I participated facilitated these Survival Trips at Payson High for about eight years, running two or three trips a year. Gary grew the program across the district in all the schools and ran the trips for several years after I left. My doctoral dissertation was based on these trips, and we really did find that the students increased in self-concept as well as in appreciation for their families during those short interventions. And…. our program did impact the dropout rate in the district.

At that time we would typically have three school staff and maybe an intern with thirty students (scary ratio, right?). The good news is that they had all elected to come. In fact, they had to get permission from their teachers to be allowed to come, so we had a very motivated crew… no AWOLS here. But it makes me shudder as I remember…we were in really inaccessible country with no means of communication with the outside world. Satellite phones and cell phones had not been invented. We were totally self-supported. No back-up staff. If someone got hurt, we just hiked him out. It helped that these were just 6-day trips, but in the 8 years I helped with the program, we never had a serious illness or injury.

When Doug Nelson contacted me in 1988 with the idea of a longer, more therapeutic wilderness program, I had completed my Ph.D. and was licensed as both a Psychologist and Marriage and Family Therapist. I had taken multiple classes from Doug, including the 28-day Boulder Outdoor Survival School course and the 28-day BYU survival course he held in Mexico. It didn't take any convincing for me to realize that this was a great idea. He had been doing programming for Steve Cartisano and he had some major concerns about the safety and effectiveness of Steve's program. But he saw the value in a longer intervention that allowed for more change and growth in the youth. He was also absolutely sure that what was needed in conjunction with the wilderness experiences was a strong clinical component. I was onboard immediately, and we created The Achievement Foundation: Wilderness Academy. Prior to becoming a high school counselor, I was a teacher, so I was in charge of both the educational and clinical components of the program. We launched our first group in the spring of 1989, and I was scrambling to stay ahead of the instructors with curriculum and clinical interventions. Our manuals were literally cut and pasted pages that I would run to the copy center before heading to the field. David Wescott, owner of BOSS helped me with a lot of the handbooks, and we used his staff for the first group in our primitive skills section.

As the psychologist, I insisted that we do a full psychological evaluation on each client and then often I would administer a post-course MMPI to track changes (my version of trying to do research). We didn't have the resources to make it a formal study, but I saw good things happening with the clients, which was verified in their post-tests.

For me, personally, it was a challenge. I was married and had two small children, daughters, ages 4 and 2. And as fate would have it, I found I was pregnant with our third daughter in the spring of 1989. When I went to the field to do therapy, I would bring a baby-sitter with me. We would set up camp near the student camp. Then I would hike in to see the clients while my little ones played in the desert. It worked out ok, and they have a love of camping that continues today. When winter came, it got harder. I had to leave them with baby-sitters and after I had my third baby, I would take her with me... drive 3 hours from my home to the field office, feed her and leave her with a sitter in Loa, go do therapy and return in the evening, feed her, and drive back home. Obviously this was not sustainable, and when a group of investors who would eventually re-name the program the Aspen Achievement Foundation, offered to buy us out, I had to make a choice between my family and wilderness therapy. I chose my family, and it was a good thing because just one year later I had twin girls.

Fast forward to 2003. I had been doing psychological evaluations for the Division of Youth Corrections and a contract came up asking for a short-term (45-day) intensive, early intervention/diversion program for probation level teens. With some friends, we put together all the elements we thought worked for youth: wilderness, meaningful work, and the care of animals...and The Journey, LLC was born. Our start-up crew, who are still with us, are Tyler Patching, our current CEO, Chelsea Thomas, our Clinical Coordinator, and Jake Smith, our Risk Manager. We used the format from my old school trips, a 6-day Trek for part of the 45 days, and the rest of the time was spent working on ranch/farm, building fence, caring for animals, milking the cow, shoveling manure, riding the horses, and doing a shortened school day in the evening. The program was successful and helped kids from tough city neighborhoods experience the wilderness and ranch-life while learning that they were worthwhile and could be successful back home. From there, The Journey grew into several group homes and foster care programs, all using wilderness as part of the treatment milieu.

The Journey Wilderness program started in 2012 when we decided to enter the parent choice arena and use the expertise we had gained taking state-placed clients on treks to develop a full wilderness therapy program. We are still small in this platform, but continue to grow while maintaining our state funded programs. We continue to find that wilderness helps kids change!

Chapter 28

2012: Legacy Outdoor Adventures

Gil Hallows

http://www.legacyoutdooradventures.com

THE SPRING EQUINOX OF 2011 IS ONE I WILL never forget. I had been summoned to a meeting in Salt Lake City by my supervisor at CRC Health Group, the company that owned the two wilderness programs I oversaw, Aspen Achievement Academy (AAA) and Passages to Recovery (PTR), located in Loa, Utah. Many private-pay programs had experienced a decline in profitability as a result of the recession, including the two programs in Loa under my directorship but I had recently told my staff teams that we were out of the woods and had survived the recession. So there I was sitting in a small meeting room with several other executive directors representing other CRC programs who were about to hear the same solemn news. Imagine my surprise when a corporate representative started the meeting by placing a box of tissue on the table, and turning to me, said, "Gil, we're going to close your programs."

During the next few minutes, I quickly cycled through the initial shock of the surprising and tragic news and into the anger phase (How, please tell me, I demanded, do you close two programs that have been as influential and profoundly impactful on so many lives as AAA and PTR?). At my first opportunity, I stepped into the hall and called my wife Flora to relay the sad development to her. Before I could finish telling her what had just happened, she interrupted to say, "You're going to start a program, aren't you?"

Returning to Loa the following day, the first item of business was delivering the bombshell to the AAA and PTR teams, whose predictable reactions of shock and anger paralleled my own. The second item of business was to begin the painful process of determining who would stay on to finish out our current clients and close the programs down, and who would be laid off immediately. The team members had poured themselves over the years and decades into creating two quality "built to last" programs, and felt a powerful and deserved sense of ownership. There followed much grieving which eventually evolved into a celebration of what we had built together, and that we were now bringing to an end.

I immediately began considering prospective partners to invite to join with me in starting the new program. I invited Troy Faddis, AAA Clinical Director, Larry Bray, AAA Program Director, and Ray Barlow, PTR Program Director to a late evening meeting, laid out what I had in mind, and invited them to join me. These were leaders with whom I had worked for many years, whose work ethic and competencies were exceptional, and who would now help create and carry out a shared vision. For the next five months that it took to graduate our last clients from AAA and PTR, we would continue to perform our duties for our employer, while assembling at night in an off-site location to envision and create the new program.

The first decision we collectively made was that we were going to start the program by pooling our modest financial resources, relying heavily on the sweat equity of the partners and the willingness of our first employees to work at temporarily reduced salaries, and pull this off with no outside investment. We were resolved to create an organization where there would be no decision-making power by anyone other than those of us who were sitting in the dirt with our clients. It was a huge risk, but having recently experienced the downside of decisions made in board rooms by people who are far removed from the work on the ground, it was a risk we were willing to take.

We then faced the bitter-sweet task of hand picking the small number of staff we would need for the startup. It was difficult to tell so many good people who wanted to work with us at the new program that we did not have a position for them. On the other hand, we enjoyed the luxury of selecting an all-star team from a large roster of supremely-qualified candidates.

Legacy Outdoor Adventures enjoyed several other advantages that many startups do not have. We did not even consider moving out of Loa. It is where we had chosen to live, our families were rooted here, and it is a great place to run a wilderness program. The closure of the previous programs created an opportunity to move right in to the land-use permits that had been vacated by the closures and apply for them under the new company. We had long-standing working relationships with the Forest Service, Bureau of Land Management and state land management agencies, and they welcomed us acquiring the vacated permits. We were approached by county officials, concerned about losing the community's largest employer, who asked what they could do to support us in creating jobs. They offered an empty office building, deferring rent payments until we got on our feet financially.

We now found ourselves in the liberated position of having the opportunity to create our ideal program, with no higher authority having to approve. We could draw from our vast collective experience in wilderness programming to pull forward those components that we knew to be effective, while capitalizing on the fresh start to incorporate some innovations. Because we intended to stay small scale, we opted to define the population we served as young adult males struggling with substance abuse and co-occurring mental health issues. We deemed it crucial to retain the fundamental parts of the basic and profoundly impactful wilderness experience, with its built-in "Hero's Journey. Within the framework of the wilderness expedition, we would incorporate a hefty component of adventure, utilizing such readily-available adventures as canyoneering, rappelling, climbing, mountain biking and fishing, with the intent of drawing our clients into their own experience and maximizing therapeutic benefits.

Landing on a name for the program took months. None of the many suggestions got any lasting traction until one day we were pondering the question of how our name needed to encapsulate the significant legacy represented by AAA and PTR within the entire field of wilderness therapy, and the far-reaching influence that the small town of Loa had bestowed on the many people who had experienced profound journeys of self-discovery here as students or employees. We all paused and looked at each other, and "Legacy" emerged as if by group think. One of the partners later proposed adding Outdoor Adventures, which, not completely by chance, results in the acronym LOA.

The net product of our intensive envisioning and planning process is a core ideology that we have come to call our "Legacy Way of Being." Our core is built around a compassionate approach to dealing with our clients and each other, strongly influenced by The Arbinger Institute, which we call having a "heart at peace." We round out our core with the concepts of honorable manhood, self-awareness, and recovery, and define each as a way of being. Our curriculum, with the "Life Success Plan" as the base, is designed to support our clients developing a vision of and progressing toward an honorable, self-aware, sober and compassionate way of living. We have set about creating an intentional community where we invite prospective new employees to get a look at our core ideology and how we deliver a wilderness therapy experience to our clients before deciding to choose in.

Even though facilitating the closing of two wilderness programs that had touched the lives of thousands was excruciatingly painful, I quickly came to see that it was only through the closing of that chapter that a new chapter could begin. The opening of the new chapter has been accompanied by an upswelling of energy, excitement and hope. Pulling a team together and creating Legacy has been without a doubt the most fulfilling accomplishment in my professional life.

Chapter 29

2014 The Making of Evoke Therapy Programs

Rick Heizer

http://evoketherapy.com

After 15 years operating as one principal company, Second Nature arrived at a collective crossroads. It became clear among the owners there was a division on the direction of the partnership and an overall difference in vision. In 2014, Second Nature partners Brad Reedy, Matt Hoag, Rick Heizer, J. Huffine, and Michael Griffin separated and became the sole owners of Second Nature Entrada and Second Nature Cascades. This separation allowed the new ownership of Second Nature Entrada and Second Nature Cascades to realize their vision, and they became Evoke Therapy Programs.

More than a name change, Evoke was a complete change in philosophy and identity. This new vision embraced an internally healthy community, where significant change and inspiration started within each owner and employee and authentically spread to the participants in the field. This concept shifted the viewpoint from a programmatic emphasis to an individually focused experience, evoking lasting change in participants through discovering the truth and wisdom found *within* the individual. The name Evoke was chosen out of a deep respect for the clients they worked with, that it wasn't the therapists' or instructors' expertise in providing advice that created change, but their ability to create the experience of self-discovery and draw out that enduring source of truth from each individual client.

The extensive and exciting experience of rebranding Entrada and Cascades was directed by the ownership with Melanie Lynch, Leah

Halverson, Steve Kirk and Stephanie Lewis playing key roles. Evoke would continue to provide high levels of clinical care, family support and active research, led by Research Director Katie Massey and Matt Hoag. Evoke would also incorporate a greater focus on whole-health treatment for their participants, families and employees. Their collaborative effort resulted in a name they felt powerfully represented their new company, as well as a logo and brand that retained the positive values of Second Nature while incorporating their new, innovative and progressive ideals.

The Evoke owners knew real growth and innovation grows from the ground level and turned their gaze inward. They made one of their founding principles a commitment to their organizational health. This meant a continual challenge to themselves and employees to create an environment of cohesion, personal and professional growth and collective support. Through regular work and recreational retreats like company river rafting and canyoneering trips, Evoke employees are able to remain accountable to this commitment. Evoke provides full and subsidized funding for all sorts of whole health activities related to the employee's mind, body and soul, such as college tuition support, gym memberships, professional development conferences, spiritual and mental health retreats, and extended vacations and sabbaticals, to name a few. The owners lead by example through regular attendance in personal growth programs and conferences.

Another way Evoke supported their mission of organizational health was to continue to organize and facilitate the Forum of Innovated Treatment Solutions (FITS) conference and bring together influential and role-modeling professionals from within and outside of their field. An annual forum, FITS is an educational, collaborative and experiential symposium in which Evoke brings together leaders in the treatment community to improve treatment outcomes in the areas of mental health and addiction. The net result of this collaboration is clients being provided with greater options, better services, and improved overall treatment outcomes due to the collaboration and discovery by the professionals themselves.

Evoke also incorporated a greater focus on their whole-health treatment, which includes the client's emotional, mental, physical, and spiritual wellbeing. This focus incorporates the clinical research which shows that diet, nutrition, exercise and spiritual connection enhances and maintains positive psychological changes, elevates moods and increases confidence. Overhauling their existing programming to incorporate greater whole health treatment became one of the larger undertakings for Evoke. Decisive collaboration was imperative to make this happen and was fulfilled by Rick Heizer, Elise Mitchell, Josh Nelson, Katelyn Bevard, Katie Rehani, and Jon Baker. The entire Evoke clinical team also played significant roles in recreating Evoke's programming, known in the field as The Journey Packet. Key clinical contributors included Lauren Roberts, Sean Roberts, Mayer Jeppson, Paul Goddard, Peter Allen, Sabrina Hadeed, David Johnson, Caitlin Tharaldson, Mike Mein, Cassidy Miller, Birgit Show, John Tobias and Josh Larson.

Family Support continued to be a primary focus for Evoke, providing weekly, live, interactive, psycho-educational webinars, parent support groups, and workshops; Evoke also made an increased investment in parent and family work and created new programming to generate larger impacts of change in the lives of their clients and families. Evoke's Heroic Journeys are multi-day intensives for individuals, parents and families to confront their own dilemmas and find greater balance, peace and clarity. Evoke's extensive family programming and support had its major contributors as well; through the leadership of Brad Reedy, with Gail Bramlet, Mischa Shriver, Jesi Gorzalski, and Lindsey Bosse played essential roles in establishing extensive programming and procedures in supporting the families of Evoke. Additional contributions were made by those who provide constant support and communication, including our medical staff; Adam Garrard, Jessica Oddo and Clint Atkinson. Evoke's commitment to create innovative comprehensive programming led them to specialized groups like their 12-Step recovery programming, adolescent adventure activities, and Pursuits. Pursuits are adventure trips providing leadership, communication and technical skills in outdoor adventure activities like canyoneering, rock climbing and river rafting that provide participants with greater self-confidence and a deeper understanding of their own personal journey.

Beyond Evoke's pledge to its organizational health, what makes Evoke unique today will likely not be what makes it unique tomorrow. With the continued commitment to evolve with new challenges and ideas, to constantly be innovative with the contributions from employees, and a dedication to the authenticity to our process of change, those are the things that will define what continues to make Evoke Therapy Programs unique.

Did you enjoy reading Stories from the Field? If so, we would appreciate it if you could please post a review on Amazon. Thank you.

Here are links to both the print and kindle editions:

Kindle edition:
http://bit.ly/storiesfromthefieldkindle

Print edition:
http://bit.ly/storiesfromthefieldpaperback

If you'd like to join our mailing list please send us an email at:
wild@wildernesspublishers.com

Epilogue

While working on this book, I have experienced that history marches on without care for the writer. Once I have something ready to print some of the story changes. Some current examples are the Boy Scouts of America are now willing to have gay or lesbian volunteers, the majority of OBH member programs are now accredited by AEE, and some of the people mentioned in Part II of this book are no longer associated with their programs that they are mentioned in. However, as of late August 2015, all programs discussed in Part II of this book are still operating, serving thousands of young people and their families through wilderness therapy.

In Part I of this book one can see that the wilderness therapy field is not perfect and some of its practitioners have harmed the families that they professed to serve. To those who have been have been harmed by this field,that I believe so much in, I am deeply sorry. There are no excuses in harming others in the name of helping. It is our duty, as practitioners and believers in wilderness therapy to be ever vigilant with our own practices and to remain open to feedback from critics, both internally and externally, as without that we can be blind to our own filters.

What is inspiring for me, to see in this time in the evolution of the field, is a greater emphasis on research, evidenced-based practices, standards of care and external oversight. I am optimistic about this continuing trend and for the future of this field.

My hope is to publish a new edition of this book in several years to continue to tell the stories of this ever-evolving field of healthcare.

Will White
August, 2015

Bibliography of Research in Outdoor Behavioral Healthcare, Adventure and Wilderness Therapy

Bettman, J., Tucker, A., Tracy, J., & Parry, K. (2014). An exploration of gender, client history and functioning in wilderness therapy participants. *Residential Treatment for Children and Youth,* 31(3), 155-170. doi:10.1080/0886571X.2014.943554.

Bowen, D., & Neill, J. (2013). A meta-analysis of adventure therapy outcomes and moderators. *The Open Psychology Journal,* 6, 28-53.

Gass, M. A., Gillis, H. L., & Russell, K. C. (2012). *Adventure therapy: Theory, research, and practice.* New York: Routledge/Taylor & Francis Group.

Gillis, H.L., Gass, M.A., & Russell, K.C. (2014). Adventure therapy with groups. In J. DeLucia Waack, C. Kalodner, & M. Riva (Eds), *The handbook of group counseling and psychotherapy* (2nd Ed.)(pp. 560-570). Thousands Oaks, CA: Sage Publications.

Norton, C.L. (2011). Wilderness therapy: Creating a context of hope. In C.L. Norton (Ed.), *Innovative interventions in child and adolescent mental health* (pp. 66-140). New York: Routledge.

Norton, C.L. (2013). Creating group norms around the campfire: Adventure based group work with adolescents. In L. Grobman & J. Clements (Eds.), *Riding the mutual aid bus and other adventures in group work: A Days in the Lives of Social Workers collection.* Harrisburg, PA: The New Social Worker

Norton, C.L., Carpenter, C. & Pryor, A. (2015). *Adventure therapy around the globe: International perspectives and diverse approaches.* Champaign, IL: Common Ground Publishing.

Norton, C.L., Tucker, A., Russell, K.C, Bettman, J., Gass, M., Gillis, L, & Behrens, E. (2014). Adventure therapy with youth. Journal of Experiential Education, 37(1), 46 - 59. doi:10.1177/1053825913518895.

Russell, K. C. (2000). Exploring how the wilderness therapy process relates to outcomes. *Journal of Experiential Education,* 23, 170-176.

Russell, K. C. (2001). What is wilderness therapy? *Journal of Experiential Education,* 24, 70- 79.

Russell, K. C. (2003). A nation-wide survey of outdoor behavioral healthcare programs for adolescents with problem behaviors. *Journal of Experiential Education,* 25, 322-331.

Russell, K. C. (2006). Brat camps, boot camps, or....? Exploring wilderness therapy program theory. *Journal of Adventure Education and Outdoor Learning,* 6, 51-67.

Russell, K. C., Gillis, H. L., & Lewis, T. G. (2008). A five-year follow-up of a nationwide survey of outdoor behavioral healthcare programs. *Journal of Experiential Education,* 31, 55-77.

Tucker, A. R. (2009). Adventure-based group therapy to promote social skills in adolescents. *Social Work with Groups,* 32(4), 315-329.

Tucker, A., Norton, C., Itin, C., Hobson, J. & Alvarez, M.A. (in press). Adventure therapy: Non deliberative group therapy in action, *Social Work with Groups*

OBH's Impact on Mental Health in Youth

Bettman, J., Clarkson Freeman, P., & Parry, K., (2015 – Online First). Differences between adopted and non-adopted adolescents in wilderness and residential treatment. *The Journal of Experiential Education.* doi:10.1177/1053825915569056

Bettman, J.E., Russell, K.C., & Parry, K.J. (2012). How substance abuse recovery skills, readiness to change and symptom reduction impact change processes in wilderness therapy participants. *Journal of Child and Family Studies,* 22(8), 1039-1050. doi:10.1007/s10826-012-9665-2

DeMille, S. M. & Burdict, M. (2015). A theoretically anchored and multi-modal treatment approach in an Outdoor Behavioral Healthcare program. *Journal of Therapeutic Schools and Programs,* 7, 19-30.

Lewis, S. F. (2013). Examining changes in substance use and conduct problems among treatment-seeking adolescents. *Child and Adolescent Mental Health,* 18(1), 33-38.

Magle-Haberek, N., Tucker, A., & Gass, M. (2012). The effects of program differences within wilderness therapy and residential treatment center (RTC) programs. *Residential Treatment for Children and Youth,* 29(3), 202-218. doi:10.1080/0886571X.2012.697433

Massey, K., Hoag, M., Roberts, S., & Javorski, S. (In Press). A multilevel model to examine adolescen outcomes in Outdoor Behavioral Healthcare: The parent perspective. *Child and Youth Care Forum.*

Norton, C.L. (2008). Understanding the impact of wilderness therapy on adolescent depression and psychosocial development. *Illinois Child Welfare,* 4(1), 166-178.

Norton, C.L. (2010). Into the wilderness – A case study: The psychodynamics of adolescent depression and the need for a holistic intervention. *Clinical Social Work Journal,* 38(2), 226-235. doi:10.1007/s10615-009-0205-5.

Norton, C.L. (2010). Exploring the process of a therapeutic wilderness experience: Key therapeutic components in the treatment of adolescent depression and psychosocial development. *Journal of Therapeutic School and Program,* 4(1), 24-46.

Russell, K. C. (2002). Does outdoor behavioral healthcare work? A review of studies on the effectiveness of OBH as an intervention and treatment. *Journal of Therapeutic Camping, Summer/Fall,* 2, 5-12.

Russell, K. C. (2003). Assessing treatment outcomes in outdoor behavioral healthcare using the Youth Questionnaire. *Child and Youth Care Forum,* 32, 355-381.

Russell, K. C. (2005). Preliminary results of a study examining the effects of outdoor behavioral healthcare treatment on levels of depression and substance use frequency. *Journal of Experiential Education,* 27, 305-307.

Russell, K. C. (2005). Two years later: A qualitative assessment of youth-well-being and the role of aftercare in outdoor behavioral healthcare treatment. *Child and Youth Care Forum,* 34, 209-239.

Russell, K. C. (2008). Adolescent substance-use treatment: Service delivery, research on effectiveness, and emerging treatment alternatives. Journal of Groups in Addiction & Recovery, 2(2-4), 68-96.

Russell, K. C., & Farnum, J. (2004). A concurrent model of the wilderness therapy process. *Journal of Adventure Education and Outdoor Learning,* 4, 39-55.

Russell, K. C., & Phillips-Miller, D. (2002). Perspectives on the wilderness therapy process and its relation to outcome. *Child and Youth Care Forum,* 31, 415-437.

Russell, K. C., & Sibthorp, J. (2004). Hierarchical linear modeling of treatment outcomes in outdoor behavioral healthcare. *Journal of Experiential Education,* 27, 176-191.

Tucker, A., Smith, A., & Gass, M. (2014). The impact of presenting problems and individual client characteristics on treatment outcomes in residential and wilderness treatment programs. *Residential Treatment for Children and Youth,* 31(2), 135-153.

Tucker, A. R., Zelov, R., & Young, M. (2011). Four years along: Emerging traits of programs in the NATSAP Practice Research Network (PRN). *Journal of Therapeutic Schools and Programs,* 5(1), 10-28.

White, D. D., Caulkins, M., & Russell, K. C. (2006). The role of physical exercise in wilderness therapy for troubled adolescent women. *Journal of Experiential Education,* 29, 18-37.

Zelov, R., Tucker, A. R., & Javorksi, S. (2013). A new phase for the NATSAP PRN: Post-discharge reporting and transition to the network wide utilization of the Y-OQ 2.0. *Journal of Therapeutic Schools & Programs,* 6(1), 7-19.

OBH's Impact on Mental Health in Young Adults

Hoag, M. J., Massey, K. M., & Roberts, S. (2014). Dissecting the wilderness therapy client: Examining clinical trends, findings, and industry patterns. *Journal of Experiential Education,* 37(4), 382-396.

Hoag, M. J., Massey, K. E., & Roberts, S. D., & Logan, P. (2013). Efficacy of wilderness therapy for young adults: A first look. *Journal of Residential Treatment for Children and Youth,* 30, 294-305.

Russell, K. C., Gillis, H. L., & Heppner, W. (In press). An examination of mindfulness-based Experience through adventure in substance use disorder treatment for young adult males: A Pilot Study. *Mindfulness.*

Attachment and OBH

Bettman, J.E. (2007). Changes in adolescent attachment relationships as a response to wilderness treatment. *Journal of the American Psychoanalytic Association,* 55 (1), 259-265

Bettman, J.E, Demong, E., & Jasperson, R.A. (2008). Treating adolescents with attachment and adoption issues in wilderness therapy settings. *Journal of Therapeutic Schools and Programs,* 8(1), 117-138.

Bettman, J.E., & Jasperson, R.A. (2008). Adults in wilderness treatment: A unique application of attachment theory and research. *Clinical Social Work Journal,* 36 (1), 51-61.

Bettman, J.E., Lundahl, B.W., Wright, R.A., Jasperson, R.A., & McRoberts, C. (2011). Who are they? A descriptive study of adolescents in wilderness and residential programs. *Residential Treatment for Children and Youth,* 28 (3), 198-210.

Bettman, J.E, Olson-Morrison, D., & Jasperson, R.A. (2011). Adolescents in wilderness treatment: A qualitative study of attachment relationships. *Journal of Experiential Education,* 34 (2), 176-194.

Bettman, J. & Tucker, A. (2011). Shifts in attachment relationships: A study of adolescents in wilderness treatment. *Child and Youth Care Forum,* 40(6), 499-519. doi:10.1007/s10566-011-9146-6

OBH's Impact on Physical Health

Tucker, A., Norton, C., DeMille, S., & Hobson, J. (in press). The impact of wilderness therapy on physical and emotional health: Utilizing an integrated approach in Outdoor Behavioral Healthcare. Journal of Experiential Education.

DeMille, S., Comart, C., & Tucker, A. (2014). Body composition changes in an Outdoor Behavioral Healthcare program. Ecopsychology, 6(3), 174-182.

Family and OBH

Faddis, T.J. & Bettman, J.E. (2006). Reflecting team and other innovative family therapy techniques, adapted for outdoor behavioral mental health settings. *Journal of Therapeutic Schools and Programs,* 1, 57-69.

Harper, N. & Russell, K. C. (2008). Family involvement and outcome in adolescent wilderness treatment: A mixed-methods evaluation. *International Journal of Child and Family Welfare, 1,* 19-36.

Harper, N., Russell, K. C., & Cooley, R. (2006). An exploratory examination of changes in adolescent and family well-being following a wilderness therapy intervention. *Journal of Experiential Education, 29,* 393-396.

Harper, N., Russell, K. C., Cooley, R. & Cupples, J. (2007). Catherine Freer Wilderness Therapy Expeditions: An exploratory case study of adolescent wilderness therapy, family functioning, and the maintenance of change. *Child and Youth Care Forum, 36,* 111-129.

OBH and Juvenile Justice

Gillis, H. L. & Gass, M. A. (2010). Treating juveniles in a sex offender program using adventure-based programming: A matched group design. *Journal of Child Sexual Abuse,* 19(1), 20-34. doi:10.1080/10538710903485583

Gillis, H. L.; Gass, M. & Russell, K. C. (2008). The effectiveness of Project Adventure's behavior management program for male offenders in residential treatment. *Residential Treatment for Children and Youth, 25,* 227-247.

Russell, K. C. (2006). Evaluating the effects of the Wendigo Lake Expedition program for young offenders. *Journal of Juvenile Justice and Youth Violence, 4,* 185-203.

Walsh, M. & Russell. K. C. (2011). An exploratory study of a wilderness adventure program for young offenders. *Ecopsychology,* 2, 211-229.

Risk Management in OBH

Gass, M., & Javorski, S. (2013). 10-year incident monitoring trends in Outdoor Behavioral Healthcare: Lessons learned and future directions. Journal of Therapeutic Schools and Programs, 6, 113-129.

Russell, K. C. & Harper, N. (2006). Incident monitoring in outdoor behavioral healthcare programs: A 4-year summary of restraint, runaway, injury, and illness rates. *Journal of Therapeutic Schools and Programs,* 1, 70-90.

OBH and Transport/Escort Use

Tucker, A., Bettman, J., Norton, C.L., & Comart, C. (2015- Online First). The role of transport use in Adolescent wilderness treatment: Its relationship to readiness to change and outcome. *Child and Youth Care Forum.* doi 10.1007/s10566-015-9301-6

Community Based Applications of OBH/Adventure Therapy

Koperski, H., Tucker, A., Lung, D.M., & Gass, M. (2015). The impact of community based adventure therapy programming on stress and coping skills in adults. Practitioner Scholar: *Journal of Counseling and Professional Psychology,* 4(1), 1-16.

Norton, C.L., Watt, T., & Penn, A. (2014). Exploring the impact of a wilderness-based positive youth development program for urban youth. Journal of Experiential Education, 37(4), 335-350. doi:10.1177/1053825913503113

Tucker, A., Javorski, S., Tracy, J. & Beale, B. (2013). The use of adventure therapy in community-based mental health: Decreases in problem severity among youth clients. *Child and Youth Care Forum,* 42(2), 155-179. doi:10.1007/s10566-012-9190-x

Tucker, A. R., Sugerman, D., & Zelov, R. (2013). On Belay: Providing connection, support and empowerment to children whose parents have cancer. *Journal of Experiential Education,* 36(2) 93–105. doi:10.1177/1053825913487889

Training, Staffing & Supervision

Gass, M. A. & Gillis, H. L. (2010). ENHANCES: Adventure therapy supervision. Journal of Experiential Education, 33(1), 72-89.

Marchand, G. & Russell, K. C. (2011). Initial training of field instructors in Outdoor Behavioral Healthcare programs. *Journal of Outdoor Recreation, Education, and Leadership,* 3, 9-12.

Marchand, G. Russell, K. C. & Cross, R. (2009). An empirical examination of outdoor behavioral healthcare field instructor job related stress and retention. *Journal of Experiential Education,* 31, 359-375.

Norton, C.L. (2012). Supervision in adventure therapy: Building something with that. In M. Gass, H.L. Gillis, & K.C. Russell (Eds.), *Adventure therapy.* New York: Routledge.

Norton, C. L., & Tucker, A. R. (2010). New heights: Adventure-based group work in social work education & practice. *Groupwork,* 20(2), 24-44.

Tucker, A. R., & Norton, C.L. (2013). The use of adventure therapy techniques by clinical social workers: Implications for practice and training. Clinical Social Work Journal, 41, 333–343. doi:10.1007/s10615-012-0411-4

Additional Publications

Gillis, H L. & Speelman. E.(2008). Are Challenge (Ropes) Courses an Effective Tool? A Meta-Analysis. *The Journal of Experiential Education,* 31(2), 111-135.

Norton, C.L. & Hsieh, C. (2011). Cultural bridging through shared adventure: Cross cultural perspectives in adventure therapy. *Journal of Adventure Education and Outdoor Learning,* 11(2), 173-188.

Norton, C.L., Wisner, B., Krugh, M., Penn, A. (2014). Helping youth transition into an alternative residential school setting: Exploring the effects of a wilderness orientation program on youth purpose and identity complexity. *Child and Adolescent Social Work Journal,* 31(5), 475-493

Russell, K. C. & Gillis, H. L. (2010). Experiential therapy in the mental health treatment of adolescents. *Journal of Therapeutic Schools and Programs,* 4, 47-79.

Tucker, A. R., & Rheingold, A. (2010). Enhancing fidelity in adventure education and adventure therapy. *Journal of Experiential Education,* 33(3), 258-273.

References

Adams, D. (1987). *A Path of Honor: The Story of VisionQuest.* Tucson, AZ: Blue Horse Productions.

Aspen Education Group Closes Five Programs. Retreived Janury 15, 2015, http://www.strugglingteens.com/artman/publish/ AspenEducationGroupBN_130710.shtml#sthash.0O9YvwWE. dpuf

Aspen Education Group to Restructure Programs. Retreived January, 15, 2015, (from http://www.strugglingteens.com/artman/publish/ AspenEducationGroupBN_110324.shtml).

Atkinson, R. (1998). *The Life Story Interview: Qualitative research methods series 44.* Thousand Oaks, CA: Sage.

Boulder Outdoor Survival School. (2011). *The History of Boss.* Retrieved from http://www.boss-inc.com/boss-basics_the-history-of-boss_70. html

Boy Scouts of America. (2011). *About the BSA.* Retrieved from http:// www.scouting.org/About.aspx

Boyle, P. (1994). *Scout's Honor: Sexual Abuse in Americas Most Trusted Institution.* Rocklin, CA: Prima Publishing.

Brekke, J. (2005, May 4). *Therapists in the Woods.* Retrieved from http:// www.strugglingteens.com/artman/publish/article_5124.shtml

Caplan, R. B. (1974). Early forms of camping in American mental hospitals. In T. L. Lowry (Ed.), *Camping Therapy* (pp. 8-12). Springfield, IL: Charles C Thomas.

Clandinin, D. J., & Connelly, F. M. (2000). *Narrative Inquiry.* San Francisco, CA: Jossey- Bass.

Cockerill, E., & Witmer, H. (1939). An evaluation of a psychiatric camp for children. *Smith College Studies in Social Work,* IX(3), 199-236.

Cole, E., Erdman, E., & Rothblum, E. (Eds.). (1994). *Wilderness Therapy for Women: The Power of Adventure.* New York, NY: The Haworth Press.

Cooley Retires, Catherine Freer Closes. Retrieved January, 15, 2015, http://www.strugglingteens.com/artman/publish/CatherineFreerBN_120614.shtml#sthash.CsZbnTQU.dpufCorvette, D. (1986, October 5). Annewakee abuses may be common former patients in probe tell of widespread sexual activity. *The Atlanta Journal,* p. D1.

Corvette, D. (1990, March 25). Anneewakee's almost out of the woods Center gains credibility with sweeping changes. *The Atlanta Journal Constitution,* p. D1.

Creswell, J. (2007). *Qualitative Inquiry & Research Design.* Thousand Oaks, CA: Sage.

Davis-Berman, J., & Berman, D. S. (1994). *Wilderness Therapy: Foundations, Theories and Research.* Dubuque, IA: Kendall/Hunt Publishing.

Davis-Berman, J., & Berman, D. S. (2008). *The Promise of Wilderness Therapy.* Dubuque, IA: Kendall/Hunt Publishing.

Dimock, H., & Hendry, C. (1929). *Camping and Character: A camp experiment in character education.* New York, NY: Association Press.

Eells, E. (1986). *History of Organized Camping: The First 100 Years.* Martinsville, IN: American Camping Association.

Eisen, G. (Producer). (1988, July 10). VisionQuest, *60 Minutes.* New York, NY: CBS News.

Ferguson, G. (1999). *Shouting at the Sky: Troubled Teens and the Promise of the Wild.* New York, NY: St. Martins Press.

Flavin, M. (1996). *Kurt Hahn's School and Legacy.* Wilmington, DE: The Middle Atlantic Press.

Galbraith, J. (1964). *Perceptions of effects of a therapeutic camping experience: Relationship to presence of nurse co-counselor and integration in treatment: A six-month follow-up study of emotionally disturbed boys at Camp Wediko.* (Unpublished doctoral dissertation). Boston University, Boston, MA.

Galkin, J. (1937). The treatment possibilities offered by the summer camp as a supplement to the Child Guidance Clinic. *The American Journal of Orthopsychiatry, VII*, 474-482.

Gass, M. (1993). *Adventure Therapy: Therapeutic Applications of Adventure Programming*. Dubuque, IA: Kendall Hunt.

Godfrey, R. (1980). *Outward Bound: Schools of the Possible*. Garden City, AL: Anchor Books.

Government Accounting Office. (2007, October 10). *Residential treatment programs – concerns death and abuse in certain programs for troubled youth*. Retrieved from http://www.gao.gov/new.items/d08146t.pdf

Government Accounting Office. (2008, April 24). *Residential treatment programs-selected cases of death, abuse and deceptive marketing*. Retrieved from http://www.gao.gov/ new.items/d08713t.pdf

Greenhouse, L. (2000, June 29). The Supreme Court: The New Jersey Case; Supreme Court Backs Boy Scouts in Ban of Gays from Membership. *The New York Times*, p. A1.

Gregory, G. (2000, February 12), *Deadly discipline?* Retrieved from http://www.teenliberty.org/deadly_discipline.htm

Hahn, K. (1960). *Outward Bound: Address at the Annual Meeting of the Outward Bound Trust, July, 20, 1960*. Retrieved from http://www.kurthahn.org/writings/obt1960.pdf

Jones, J. C. (2006). When the cameras are rolling. *Addiction Professional, 4*(1), 30-35.

Kelly, F. J., & Baer, D. J. (1968). *Outward Bound Schools as an Alternative to Institutionalization for Adolescent Delinquent Boys*. Boston, MA: Fandel Press.

Ketcham, C. (2007, May). A death at outward bound. *National Geographic Adventure*, pp. 49-55.

Kimball, R., & Bacon, S. B. (1993). The wilderness challenge model. In M. Gass (Ed.), *Adventure Therapy: Therapeutic Applications of Adventure Programming* (pp. 11-41). Dubuque, IA: Kendall/Hunt Publishing.

Krakauer, J. (1995, October). Loving them to death. *Outside Magazine*. Retrieved from http://www.outsideonline.com/outdoor-adventure/Loving-Them-to-Death.html?page=all

Krakauer, J. (2003). *Under the Banner of Heaven: Story of a Violent Faith.* New York, NY: Doubleday.

Krakauer, J. (2004, July 3). *A response from the author.* Retrieved from http://www.randomhouse.com/features/krakauer/response.html

Kramp, M. K. (2004). Exploring life and experience through narrative inquiry. In K. DeMarrais & S. D. Lapan (Eds.), *Foundations of Research* (pp. 31-50). Mahwah, NJ: Lawrence Erlbaum Associates.

Loughmiller, C. (1965). *Wilderness Road.* Austin, TX: Hogg Foundation for Mental Health.

Loughmiller, C. (1979). *Kids in Trouble.* Tyler, TX: Wildwood Books.

Loughmiller, C., & Loughmiller, L. (1959). *Let's go camping: Camping and Christian Growth.* Nashville, TN: Abingdon Press.

Loughmiller, C., Loughmiller, L., & Abernethy, F. E. (2002). *Big thicket legacy.* Austin, TX: University of Texas Press.

Loughmiller, C., Loughmiller, L., & Waitt, D. E. (2006). *Texas wildflowers: A field guide.* Austin, TX: University of Texas Press.

Lowry, T. P. (Ed.). (1974). *Camping therapy.* Springfield, IL: Charles C Thomas.

McNeil, E. B. (1957). The background of therapeutic camping. *Journal of Social Issues,* 13(1), 3-14.

McPeake, J. D., Kennedy, B., Grossman, J. & Beaulieu, L. (1991). Innovative adolescent chemical dependency treatment and its outcome: A model based on Outward Bound programming: *Journal of Adolescent Chemical Dependency,* 2(1), 29-57.

Medrick, F. W. (1977). Confronting passive behavior through outdoor experience: A TA approach to experiential learning. In Northeastern Forest Experiment Station (Ed.), *Children, Nature, and the Urban Environment: Proceedings of a Symposium-Fair* (pp. 192-198). Upper Darby, PA: U.S. Department of Agriculture, Forest Service.

Miner, J., & Boldt, J. (1991). *Outward Bound USA: Learning through experience in adventure-based education.* New York, NY: William Morrow & Co.

Miner, J., Boldt, J., & Eno, M. (1981). *Outward Bound USA: Crew not passengers.* Seattle, WA: Mountaineer Books.

Mitchell, V., & Crawford, I. (1950). *Camp Counseling.* Philadelphia: W.B. Saunders Co.

Morgenstern, J. (1995). *A Death in the Desert.* Retrieved from http://articles.latimes.com/
1995-01-15/magazine/tm-20285_1_private-school-public-school-gifted

Morse, W. (1947). From the University of Michigan fresh air camp: Some problems of therapeutic camping. *The Nervous Child,* 6, 211-224.

Morse, W. (1957). An interdisciplinary therapeutic camp. Journal of Social Issues, 13(1), 15-22.

Newes, S. (2000). *Adventure-based therapy: Theory, characteristics, ethics, and research.* A review of published literature through 2000. (Unpublished doctoral dissertation). Pennsylvania State University, Pennsylvania, PA.

Nold, J., & Wilpers, M. (1975). Wilderness training as an alternative to incarceration. In C. Dodge (Ed.), *A Nation Without Prisons: Alternatives to Incarceration* (pp. 155-169). Lexington, MA: Lexington Books.

Powch, G. I. (1994). Wilderness Therapy: What Makes it Empowering for Women? *Women & Therapy,* 15(4), 11-27.

Rademacher, E. S. (1928). Treatment of problem children by means of a long-term camp. *Mental Hygiene, XII,* 385-390.

Ringholz, R. C. (1998). *On Belay!: The Life of Legendary Mountaineer Paul Petzoldt.* Seattle, WA: Mountaineers Books.

Roche, L. R. (1989, August 16). Two operators helped start program but both later left because they disliked the way it was being run. *Desert News.* Retrieved from http://www.deseretnews.com/article/59781/2-OPERATORS-HELPED-START-PROGRAM.html

Rousmaniere, K. (2004). Historical research. In K. DeMarrais & S. D. Lapan (Eds.), *Foundations of research* (pp. 31-50). Mahwah, NJ: Lawrence Erlbaum Associates.

Rowan, E. L. (2005). *To Do My Best: James E. West and the History of the Boy Scouts of America.* Las Vegas, NV: Edward Rowan.

Russell, K. (2007). *Summary of research from 1999-2006 and update of 2000 survey of outdoor behavioral healthcare programs in North America.* Technical Report # 2. Minneapolis, MN: Outdoor Behavioral Research Cooperative, Minnesota.

Russell, K., & Hendee, J. (2000). *Outdoor behavioral healthcare: Definitions, common practice, expected outcomes and a nationwide* survey of programs. *Technical Report # 26.* Moscow, ID: Wilderness Research Center, University of Idaho.

Russell, K., Gillis, L. and Lewis, T.G. (2008) A Five-Year follow-up of a North American Survey of outdoor behavioral healthcare programs. *Journal of Experiential Education,* 31(1), 55-57.

Santa, J. (2007). The history of private residential treatment programs. *Journal of the National Association of Therapeutic Schools and Programs,* 2(1), 15-25.

Schutt, D. (2000, September). *Press release.* Retrieved from http://www. strugglingteens.com/news/lakectydistattorney.html

Seymour, S.R. (1976). *Outdoor wilderness survival and its psychological and sociological effects upon student in changing human behavior.* (Unpublished doctoral dissertation). Brigham Young University, Provo, UT.

Schoel, J. (1978). *Counseling on the Run: Adventure based counseling manual.* Hamilton, MA: Project Adventure.

Schoel, J., & Maizell, R. S. (2002). *Exploring the Islands of Healing.* Beverly, MA: Project Adventure.

Schoel, J., Prouty, D., & Radcliffe, P. (1988). *Islands of Healing.* Hamilton, MA: Project Adventure.

Smith, B. (1958). *The Worth of a Boy.* Austin, TX. The Hogg Foundation.

Stednitz, L. (1991, June). *Aspen Achievement Academy.* Retrieved from http://www.strugglingteens.com/archives/1991/6/oe01.html

Stich, T. F. (1983). Experiential Therapy. *Journal of Experiential Education,* 5(5), 23-30.

Sudetic, C. (2000, July 6). The Struggle for the Soul of the Boy Scouts. *Rolling Stone.* Retrieved from http://www.bsa-discrimination.org/html/rollingstone.html

Szalavitz. M. (2006). *Help at Any Cost.* New York, NY: Penguin Group.

Watson, G. B. (1928) *Some accomplishments in summer camps.* New York, NY: Associated Press.

Watts, S. T. (2003) *Better an Honest Scoundrel: Chronicle of a Western Lawman.* Victoria, Canada: Trafford Publishing.

Wells, L. (1978). *A Guide to Wilderness Therapy Programs.* Salt Lake City, UT: Self.

White, W. (2008). A mighty change: The influence of Larry Dean Olsen on the evolution of wilderness therapy. *Journal of the National Association of Therapeutic Schools and Programs,* 3(1), 8-19.

Wilson, R. A. (2007). Combining Historical Research and Narrative Inquiry to Create Chronicles and Narratives. *The Qualitative Report,* 12(1), 1-37.

Woodbury, L. (1991a). *Catherine freer wilderness survival school.* Retrieved from   http://www.strugglingteens.com/archives/1991/8/np01.html

Woodbury, L. (1991b). *Wilderness Conquest History.* Retrieved from http://www.strugglingteens.com/archives/1991/6/news01.html

Woodbury, L. (1992, April). North Star Expeditions. Retrieved from http://www.strugglingteens.com/archives/1992/4/np02.html

Zinn, H. (1997). *A People's History of the United States.* New York, NY: The New Press.

Index

T

Author Biography

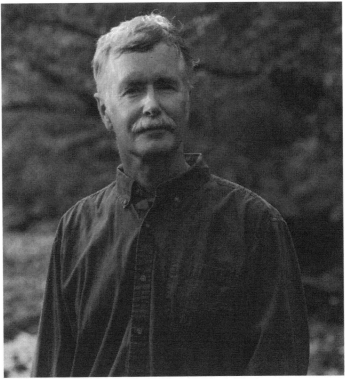

Dr. Will White received his Master of Social Work degree from the University of Denver and his Doctorate degree in Leadership from Franklin Pierce University. He has been licensed as a Clinical Social Worker and Alcohol and Drug Abuse Counselor for over 25 years.

Dr. White is co-founder of Summit Achievement. He is an nationally recognized researcher and speaker on the history of adventure and wilderness therapy. He is an adjunct professor at Plymouth State University and has served on various boards related to the field including the Therapeutic Adventure Professionals Group of the Association of Experiential Education, National Association of Therapeutic Schools and Programs and the Outdoor Behavioral Healthcare Council. His newest project is wildernespublishers.com.

He and his family live in New Hampshire.